R. Jacobs · D. van Steenberghe, Radiographic Planning and Assessment
of Endosseous Oral Implants

T0073484

Springer
Berlin
Heidelberg
New York
Barcelona
Budapest
Hong Kong
London
Milan
Paris
Santa Clara
Singapore
Tokyo

Reinhilde Jacobs · Daniel van Steenberghe

Radiographic Planning and Assessment of Endosseous Oral Implants

With 77 Figures in 145 Parts and 9 Tables

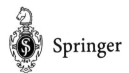 Springer

Reinhilde Jacobs, LDS, PhD, Periodontol, Postdoctoral Research Fellow of the Fund
for Scientific Research – Flanders (Belgium)
Daniel van Steenberghe, MD, PhD, Oral Surg, Periodontol, Dr hc, Holder of the P-I
Brånemark Chair in Osseointegration
Department of Periodontology
Faculty of Medicine, Catholic University of Leuven, Kapucijnenvoer 7,
B-3000 Leuven, Belgium

ISBN-13:978-3-642-80426-7

Library of Congress Cataloging-in-Publication Data

Jacobs, Reinhilde, 1967 –
Radiographic planning and assessment of endosseous oral implants /
Reinhilde Jacobs, Daniel van Steenberghe.
p. cm.
Includes bibliographical references and index.
ISBN-13:978-3-642-80426-7   e-ISBN-13:978-3-642-80424-3
DOI: 10.1007/978-3-642-80424-3
1. Endosseous dental implants-Radiography. I. Steenberghe, D. van. II. Title.
[DNLM: 1. Dental Implants. Endosseous-methods.
2. Radiography, Dental-methods. WU 640 J17r 1998] RK667-I45J3 1998
617.6'9-dc21 97-21358
DNLM/DLC
for Library of Congress

© Springer-Verlag Berlin Heidelberg 1998
Softcover reprint of the hardcover 1st edition 1998

Cover Design: Design & Production GmbH, D-69121 Heidelberg
Typesetting: FotoSatz Pfeifer GmbH, D-82166 Gräfelfing
SPIN: 10567313   24/3135 – 5 4 3 2 1 0 – Printed on acid-free paper

Preface

For several decades now, clinicians have been striving to optimise the surgical techniques for placing implants into the jaw bone. The introduction of many implant systems has been characterised by a trial and error approach. Only a few of these systems have been scientifically documented by animal experiments and long-term clinical follow-up studies. Several handbooks are dealing with the scientific basis and/or clinical application of oral implants.

Through recent developments in radiology and new insights in implant treatment, a gap exists between the available technology and clinical practice. This handbook intends to bridge this gap, providing clinical guidelines and practical information to specialists and referring dentists involved in oral implant treatment. It is meant to be a guide for radiographic planning and follow-up of oral implants, independent of the hardwares used. The book attempts to critically evaluate all imaging techniques that can be used in the planning and for the assessment of oral implants.

The information provided should urge the clinician to opt for the most precise technique available in his country, taking into account the liabilities of the radiation involved. This is especially true for the radiographic examination during the planning phase. Although dentists often prefer to use chairside oral radiology, it should be considered that implant placement is not urgent and often a unique event in a patient's life. Thus, as in the rest of medicine, the patient should often be referred to the radiologist to optimise the planning.

The writing of this handbook was made possible by the efforts of many people, to whom we are most grateful. We especially wish to recognise the contribution of the members of the Department of Periodontology, in particular Annelies Adriansens, who, with a lot of enthusiasm, collected a number of illustrations and made important contributions to our research on 3-D pre-operative planning for implant placement. We are greatly indebted to the members of the Department of Radiology, especially Prof. G. Marchal, Dr. R. Hermans and Dr. M. Smet, University Hospital Leuven, Belgium, for a good clinical collaboration and for providing specialised radiographic images (CT, MRI, scintigraphy, ...) of most of our patients. We are also indebted to the Department of Electrical Engineering (ESAT), especially Prof. P. Suetens, Dr. K. Verstreken and Dr. J. Van Cleynenbreugel. For years our department experienced a fruitful co-operation with the Department of Prosthetic Dentistry headed by Prof. I. Naert. We are very grateful to Miranda Maréchal for her commitment to finalise the draft version of this book, providing innumerable valuable suggestions and corrections. Furthermore, we want to thank Dr. David Harris for the English corrections.

We are grateful to Nobel Biocare AB, Göteborg, Sweden, for sponsoring the research on 3-D images for pre-operative planning, through the Brånemark Chair in Osseointegration, held by Prof. D. van Steenberghe. Finally, we acknowledge the support of the Fund for Scientific Research (F.W.O.) – Flanders (Belgium), enabling me as a postdoctoral research fellow to continue a career devoted to research and teaching.

This handbook is dedicated to Prof. Dr. Michel Bossuyt, head of the Department of Stomatology and Maxillofacial Surgery at the Catholic University of Leuven. He introduced me in the field of oral radiology and stimulated me to continue with it after my graduation. Over the years, he quietly but strongly provided support and encouragement for my work and for this I express my deepest gratitude.

R. Jacobs

Contents

Chapter 5. Bone Quality

Chapter 6. Radiographic Assessment of Implant Complications and/or Failures

General Introduction

D. van Steenberghe

Oral endosseous implants are used to rehabilitate (partially) edentulous or more severely handicapped patients (Fig. 1). It should be recognised that loss of teeth and the subsequent involution of periodontal tissues are comparable to other forms of amputation.

A breakthrough was achieved in the sixties with the clinical introduction of the osseointegration technique by Prof. P-I. Brånemark from Gothenburg. The principle was based on a serendipitous observation, the inability to remove an optic chamber in a pure titanium holster from the bone of experimental animals. It was further tried out in a dog model and finally applied at a clinical level. After ten years of clinical experience the Gothenburg team reported its promising clinical results (Brånemark

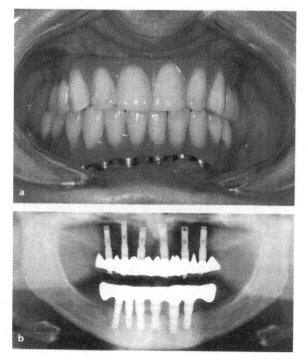

Fig. 1. Intra-oral (**a**) and radiographic (**b**) situation of an edentulous patient rehabilitated for more than 15 years with full fixed prostheses in both upper and lower jaws

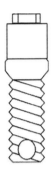

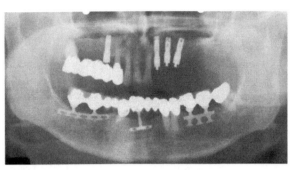

Fig. 2. Schematic presentation of a commonly used screw-shaped implant

Fig. 3. Panoramic radiograph of a patient rehabilitated with 3 different types of endosseous implants (blade-form implants, disk-form implants, screw-shaped implants)

et al. 1977). They went unnoticed until the early eighties when the 15 years report brought many researchers and clinicians in contact with Prof. Brånemark (Adell et al. 1981).

In many centres, endosseous implants, which achieve an intimate bone apposition, have been developed, mostly using a commercially pure or an alloyed titanium (Fig. 2). Several roughened surface textures have been designed in an attempt to improve bone ingrowth. A variety of surgical approaches have also been presented; either "one-stage" which means that the implant pierces throughout the mucoperiosteum from the time of installation or "two-stage" which means a healing time of several months before an abutment piece is connected to the anchoring element through a crestal incision.

A large variety of implant morphologies have been marketed (Fig. 3). While those that are inserted by means of traumatic surgery (bone heating and/or crushing) lead to fibrous encapsulation, those that are inserted very gently and under aseptic conditions achieve a predictable bone apposition. Thus the fibrously encapsulated implants need a retentive morphology; otherwise pulling forces would easily extrude them. The bone dimensions needed will therefore be larger than for screw-shaped or cylindrical implants which achieve retention through intimate bone apposition.

The few marketed implant systems that provide some clinical documentation indicate that the combination of a limited bone volume and a poor bone quality lead to less predictable bone apposition and early onset failures. There is a need for a thorough radiological assessment to evaluate these factors so as to inform the patient on his individual prospects for a successful rehabilitation by means of endosseous implants (Part I).

Once an implant is placed and becomes functional, there is a need for regular radiographic controls to evaluate the stability of its implant to bone interface and, for permucosal implants, to ensure the stability of the marginal bone level (Part II).

Part I

Radiographic Evaluation of the Areas to Be Implanted

Radiographic Evaluation of the Areas to Be Implanted

The goal of a pre-operative radiographic evaluation is to assess both quantity and quality of the jaw bone areas to be implanted. The result of the radiographic assessment can favour alternative rehabilitations, without the use of implants, if bone characteristics seem unsuitable. It will also have an influence on the choice of the implant with respect to the dimensions, location, orientation and the numbers to be placed. An important goal is to select locations with enough cortical and cancellous bone to insure a good primary stability. There are indeed arguments to postulate that a poor fixation can lead to micromovements during the healing time and dedifferentiation to scar tissue cells of the bone cells invading the space between bone and implant. Such a fibrous encapsulation is comparable to a non-union fracture which is also clearly associated with a lack of stability during the primary healing phase. The pre-operative radiographic evaluation should provide information about the height and width of the bone, the degree of corticalisation, the density of mineralisation and the amount of cancellous bone in the areas considered. Different imaging tools are available, each with strengths and weaknesses and specific indications. Clinical examination with palpation is non-invasive but provides information limited to the width and height of the jaw bone. It does not allow the assessment of critical anatomical structures such as maxillary sinuses or mandibular nerves and evidently does not provide information on other aforementioned bone parameters. Radiographic examination is therefore a necessity in the pre-operative treatment planning when endosseous implants are considered. Chapter 1 deals with the available imaging techniques, chapter 2 deals with bone quantity and quality assessment. Chapter 3 offers a practical guide for pre-operative planning of implant placement.

Chapter 1

Imaging Procedures for Pre-Operative Assessment

1.1
Introduction

Both quantitative (volume) and qualitative (e. g. degree of corticalisation) bone parameters must be assessed radiographically before the periodontologist or oral surgeon
can consider the actual placement of implants. A large variety of imaging techniques
are presently available: some have been utilised for many years; others have been made
possible by recent advances in computer technology. A distinction could also be made
between morphologic imaging to detect anatomic changes, and functional imaging to
detect physiologic changes. Morphologic imaging includes film radiography (intra-
oral, panoramic, tomographic, scanographic, stereoscopic), digital radiography (direct, indirect, subtraction), computer tomography, magnetic resonance imaging (MRI),
absorptiometry and ultrasonography. Functional imaging or radionucleide imaging
includes scintigraphy, single photon emission computer tomography (SPECT), positron
emission computer tomography (PET), thermography.

Radiographs result from exposing objects to a radiation beam with a wavelength of
10^{-1} to 10^{-3} nm. They are commonly called x-rays. A beam of x-ray photons traversing
an object is attenuated by absorption and scattering of photons. This attenuation is
dependent on the object irradiated. The x-ray photons that exit the object unaffected
carry the information and become diagnostically useful by recording on an image
receptor. The most commonly used image receptor is the x-ray film (analogue radiography). Analogue radiographs are dependent on a chemical process by interaction of
the x-ray beam with photosensitive silver bromide crystals in the film emulsion. The
chemically altered crystals constitute the latent image on the film. During the developing process the latent image is converted into a visible image. Analogue radiographic
techniques are still used by the majority of the clinicians. Digital radiography using a
CCD-sensor or phosphor plate is however becoming increasingly important.

The advantages of digital radiography are multifold:

- data can be modified at will to obtain other contrasts, magnifications, grey values
- data can be transferred by networks to distant users
- data can be displayed according to different planes in space. This reformatting
  allows the radiologist to isolate more radiosensitive tissues from the beam such as
  in imaging the oral areas
- ecological consequences are far more limited compared with analogue radiographs that depend on silver salts

In this chapter, a number of the available imaging modalities in the maxillofacial area
are discussed and their usefulness in oral implant therapy is critically assessed.

1.2.
Analogue Intra-Oral Radiography

Intra-oral radiographs allow evaluation of the remaining teeth and jaw bone in the mesiodistal dimension. Only the parallel technique should be recommended, preferably with special positioning devices and a long-cone (Fig. 1.1). This technique offers a number of advantages compared to the bisecting-angle technique:

- no image enlargement
- no image distortion
- decreased radiation dose because of the collimation

The intra-oral radiography by means of the paralleling technique reveals even minute pathological changes of the periodontium and the teeth. Such pathologies could interfere with the placement of implants and should therefore be dealt with.

It should be stressed that the placement of intra-oral films in the edentulous patient usually presents problems. The technique is difficult to accomplish in edentulous regions because of the extent of bone resorption and since the positioning device cannot be supported by remaining teeth. The film can seldom be kept parallel to the alveolar process, especially in the anterior regions of the jaw. Any valid assessment of the vertical bone dimensions becomes impossible.

The intra-oral radiograph is a two-dimensional image and does not reveal information of the vestibulo-oral dimension. Intra-oral inspection can only roughly estimate the amount of available bone. The surgeon will have to wait for the per-operative assessment of the width of the jaw bone and take the risk of finding a too narrow ridge.

The intra-oral technique can be suitable for implant site assessment for a single tooth replacement (Fig. 1.2). In the latter case, information on the mesiodistal dimensions is preferably obtained from clinical intra-oral measurements. One should take into account the minimal space needed for single tooth replacement. It is dependent on the diameter of the implant type used and aesthetic considerations of the prosthetic rehabilitation. In general, a minimum of 5.5 to 7 mm interdental space is required. The bone height can be radiographically determined while the vestibulo-oral dimension can be deducted from the measurement of the thickness of the muco-

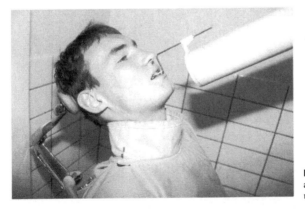

Fig. 1.1. Clinical set-up for paralleling intra-oral radiography using a long-cone

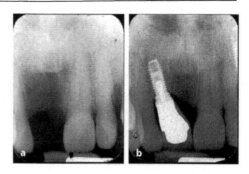

Fig. 1.2. Intra-oral radiographs of a young patient who had lost his upper central incisor. After healing of the extraction wound **(a)**, a solitary screw-shaped titanium implant was placed in this location **(b)**

periosteum both orally and labially by means of a periodontal pocket probe. Surface anaesthesia or a slight infiltration with a local anaesthetic is sufficient. The precision of such measurements is limited. The alternative, a reformatted CT (see § 1.6) seems too expensive and the radiation dose too high for such a limited rehabilitation.

Single tooth replacement is mostly performed in the frontal region where aesthetics are of primary importance. Careful considerations should be given to the implant angulation. When the pre-operative determination of the implant axis is of primary importance or when there is some doubt about the localisation or extension of adjacent anatomic structures, such as the incisive canal, a reformatted CT scan or a tomograph in the vestibulo-oral plane is recommended.

1.3.
Digital Intra-Oral Radiography

Digital radiography enables the use of computerised images which can be stored, manipulated and corrected for under- and overexposures. Digital radiography may yield almost equal image properties compared to analogue radiography, but through digital storage and processing, diagnostic information can be enhanced (Table 1.1). A digital sensor eliminates the problem associated with differences in film emulsion, developer and fixer concentrations and temperature. Certain anatomic structures can be accentuated by image manipulation. An important advantage is the dose reduction

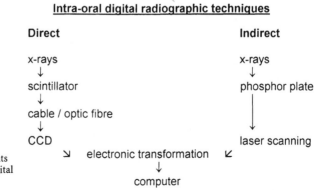

Fig. 1.3. This scheme presents both pathways to obtain digital radiography

Intra-oral digital radiographic techniques

Direct	Indirect
x-rays	x-rays
↓	↓
scintillator	phosphor plate
↓	
cable / optic fibre	
↓	↓
CCD	laser scanning

↘ electronic transformation ↙
↓
computer

Table 1.1. Advantages and disadvantages of digital radiology

	Advantages	Disadvantages	Indications
Digital radiography	• no chemicals, no dark room, no development • chairside technique • image storage • image manipulation (correction under- and overexposure) • integration in computerised patient management • communication between clinicians at different locations • radiation dose reduction	• misuse of image manipulation • lower contrast and resolution	• intraoral radiography of limited area • bone density evaluation
	direct technique • real-time	• wire • sensor rigidity • limited sensor area • no long cone RX	• endodontic treatment
	indirect technique • flexible sensor • sensor area (2 plate sizes) → conventional radiographs • wireless • use long cone possible	• manipulation and developing time	• implant follow-up

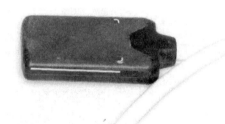

a

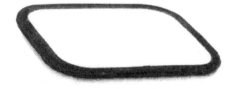

b

Fig. 1.4. a Rigid CCD sensor for the direct digital radiography. **b** Film-like sensor for the indirect digital radiography

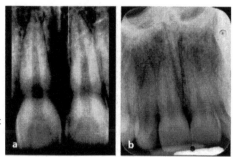

Fig. 1.5. Due to the limited sensor area of direct digital radiography **(a)**, less teeth can be depicted in comparison to conventional intra-oral radiography **(b)**

obtained with this technique. A conventional x-ray unit can be used, but dose reduction up to $1/3$ – $1/2$ is achieved when compared with the conventional intra-oral film.

Depending on the sensor, the image is presented 'direct' in real-time or 'indirect' after about half a minute of laser scanning (Fig. 1.3). In the direct technique, a Charge Coupled Device (CCD) sensor with a fibre optic or other wire is used (Fig. 1.4a). The sensor is rigid and has a limited image area (Fig. 1.5). The indirect technique utilises a phosphor plate, which is a flexible film-like radiation energy sensor (Fig. 1.4b). Photostimulable phosphor is used to store the x-ray energy, which has to be scanned by a laser beam prior to visualisation.

Digital intra-oral radiography is in a state of rapid development. Detectors as well as computer hardware and software are continually modified and improved. Different techniques are currently available for use in the dental practice (Table 1.2). Most of them render comparable results with conventional radiography (Sanderink et al. 1994; Welander et al. 1994).

The main advantage of direct digital radiography is the 'real-time' imaging, offering both the clinician and the patient an improved visualisation of the intra-oral situation by image manipulation and comparison of the actual image with previously stored ones. It has been claimed that this technique can be used per-operatively to visualise the different stages of the drill or the implant (Jeffcoat 1992a). One should however consider the necessary principles of radiation hygiene and sterility. Another advantage for pre-operative implant planning could be the evaluation of bone density

Table 1.2. Different techniques available for digital intra-oral radiography

	Company	City, Country	Sensor	Image surface (in mm²)	Time
Direct technique					
RVG	Trophy	Vincennes, France	CCD /optic fibre	30 × 20	direct
Sidexis	Siemens	Bensheim, Germany	CCD /optic fibre	29.6 × 18.4	5 sec
Flash Dent	Villa Sistemi Medicali	Buccinasco, Italy	CCD /optic fibre	variable	direct
Visualix	Gendex	Chicago, USA	CCD / cable	24.2 × 18.1	direct
Sens-A-Ray	Regam	Sundsvall, Sweden	CCD / cable	26.0 × 17.3	direct
Indirect technique					
Digora	Soredex	Helsinki, Finland	phosphor plate	40 × 30	23 s + manipulation

at the proposed implant site expressed in grey scale values which reflect the relative bone density.

Disadvantages of the direct technique are the limited sensor area (CCD), only large enough to depict an area varying from 26×17 mm^2 to 30×20 mm^2 (one or two teeth). Since dealing with a rigid sensor and wire, film positioning remains a critical factor. Special film-holders should be further developed or improved to guarantee an optimal projection geometry. Another disadvantage is that these techniques can only be used with low-voltage x-ray units. The latter implies that high-quality radiography using the long-cone paralleling technique, which requires high-voltage x-ray units cannot be achieved.

In the indirect digital radiography luminescence plates are placed intra-orally and exposed to conventional x-ray tubes. A laser scanner reads the exposed plates off-line and reveals digital image data. Advantages are that the intra-oral sensor has the size and flexibility of a standard intra-oral radiograph. The technique may also be used with all conventional x-ray tubes in contrast to the direct technique which is limited to the low voltage x-ray units. Quantitative measurements can thus be carried out when a paralleling technique is applied. It is also stated that storage phosphor systems achieve a higher image quality than CCD sensors and x-ray films (Borg and Gröndahl 1996). The presently available rigid sensor for direct digital radiography makes the evaluation of the often resorbed jaw bone difficult. The indirect technique is an improvement in this perspective because of the flexible sensor.

Considering the number of advantages, digital radiography might replace the analogue radiography in future daily practice. However, further research on the application of digital radiography is needed. Certain modifications have to be carried out to overcome the documented drawbacks such as limited sensor area and projection geometry. Only then, can this technique be considered for routine assessment of bone level and density.

1.4.
Lateral Cephalography

With regard to pre-operative planning of implant placement, the lateral cephalogram offers limited information. The structures are presented life-size and show the relationship between upper and lower jaws in the sagittal plane, but clinical examination gives the same information at no expense. The radiograph provides some information on the symphyseal area, and the inclination and bucco-lingual dimensions of the jaw bone in the anterior region. This is not very relevant when planning placement of implants since just lateral to the strict sagittal plane, anatomical concavities (sublingual) reduce the available bone volume dramatically. Furthermore, the muscular pull (m. geniohyoideus, m. genioglossus) keeps the bone loss in the strict symphyseal area to a minimum, thus creating a too optimistic bone volume assessment on lateral cephalograms. Another major disadvantage is that left and right side overlap and thus only limited information is available on the bone height. Radiation dose should be kept to a minimum by proper collimation and shielding to avoid the radiation of radiosensitive tissues. A lateral cephalogram always involves the thyroid and pituitary glands, but the collimation could limit the visualised area to the jaw bone concerned. One should check if one's apparatus allows such collimation. Occlusal films placed laterally in a vertical position at the level of the upper or lower frontal region have been suggested as an alternative (Sewerin 1991c)(Fig. 1.6).

Because of the limited diagnostic information, the use of a lateral cephalogram should be limited to those patients who need a surgical correction because of a sagittal deviation between upper and lower jaws (Fig. 1.7). In a near future, digital cephalography will become available offering similar advantages as the aforementioned digital intra-oral radiography (image manipulation, real time imaging, ...).

Furthermore, the lateral topogram (scout view) of the CT scanning images provides similar information as a conventional lateral cephalogram and makes the latter technique redundant when a CT is planned.

1.5
Panoramic Radiography

During the last few years, this technique has undergone an important evolution. It is routinely used in daily practice, especially in oral surgery. In contrast to intra-oral radiography, the position of the radiation source and the film are not static but they rotate around the patient's head. Thus, overlap of anatomic structures is partly avoided. According to Molander et al. (1995) the quality of the panoramic radiograph for different equipments is comparable. The radiation risk expressed by the effective dose varies from 6.7 to 80 µSv, with lower risk levels associated with the new equipments (Rushton and Horner 1996).

For pre-operative examinations, panoramic radiographs can be used as a screening instrument to detect pathologic changes of the teeth, the periodontium, the temporo-mandibular joints and the maxillary sinuses. It visualises the location of critical anatomic structures with a broader coverage than intra-oral radiographs. In a dentate jaw, the panoramic radiograph should be supplemented with restricted intra-oral radiographs of the dentate regions, to provide sufficient details of the latter. It remains a 2-dimensional image, lacking information on the width of the bone. The image is the product of linear tomography. The angulation of the x-ray beam is about 7 ° from below. This results in image distortion which can have serious consequences

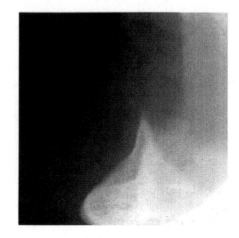

Fig. 1.6. In addition to panoramic radiography, occlusal film may be indicated to gain some information on bone width in the symphyseal region of the edentulous mandible

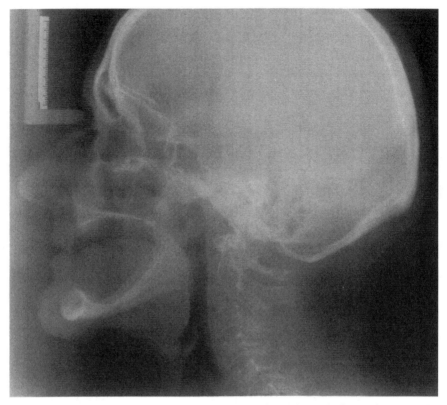

Fig. 1.7. A lateral cephalogram may be indicated in the case of severely resorbed jaws, where correction of the sagittal relationship is needed

in the assessment of the amount of bone available. Magnification occurs in both vertical and horizontal direction and varies considerably (from 1.1 to 1.3; mean 1.25–1.27) related to the positioning of the patient, and even in different areas within the same patient. This has a profound effect on the bone quantity assessment and the localisation of the anatomic structures. The magnification is more pronounced in the anterior region. The use of intensifying screens limits the resolution. All those limitations imply that the optimal implant dimensions (length and thickness) can only be roughly determined on panoramic radiographs. The identification of the mandibular canal, the floor of the maxillary sinus and the nasal fossa can be difficult and the localisation often inaccurate. It also has to be mentioned that there is a practical problem in positioning the edentulous patient within a panoramic machine in such a way that both the upper and lower jaws are placed within the focal trough as there is often an important deviation in the sagittal plane between upper and lower jaws. It is unreliable to judge the correct position in edentulous patients. Only the nasal cavity can give some help. Positioning errors in the sagittal plane result in differences in magnification, the parts closest to the film being less magnified. If the patient is placed either anterior or posterior of the desired position, an important magnification of the anterior region may occur.

For pre-operative assessment of implant placement, it can be used in the symphyseal area, taking into account local magnification and distortion (Fig. 1.8). It is helpful to use a stent or template with radiopaque markers, which might give some idea of local magnifications. Another solution, but far less accurate, is the application of an average magnification factor of 1.25–1.27.

To identify the mandibular canal the panoramic radiograph lacks precision, which can become unacceptable if the risk of damaging the nerve is present. Klinge et al.

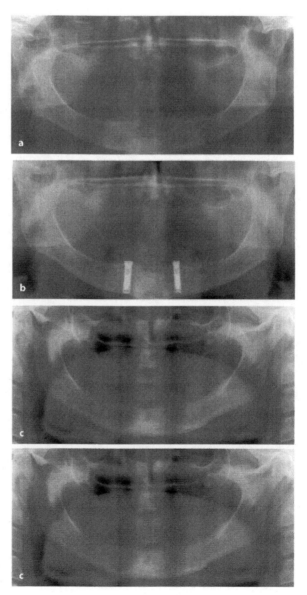

Fig. 1.8. Based on the panoramic radiograph and clinical demands of an edentulous patient **(a)**, 2 implants were placed in the symphyseal region to support an overdenture **(b)**. Based on the panoramic radiograph of another edentulous patient **(c)**, 6 implants were placed in the symphyseal region to support a full fixed prosthesis **(d)**

(1989) observed that 83 % of the bone height measurements above the canal on panoramic radiographs deviated more than 1 mm from the true value! Sonick et al. (1994) confirmed that measurements on panoramic radiographs are unreliable. They found an average amount of distortion of no less than 3 mm! In the anterior mandible in between the foramina mentales, one may assume that bone quality and quantity are sufficient for implant placement and that there is only a minor risk of interference with the nerves (Jemt et al. 1996). One should however take into account that whenever the radiographic bone height is less than 10 mm in the symphyseal area, even there, more detailed information on bone height and bucco-lingual dimension is recommended by means of specialised imaging technique (e.g. CT; Lam et al. 1995).

Finally, digital panoramic radiography in its present form has the same advantages as digital radiography in general (real time imaging, image storage and manipulation, …). The radiation dose remains however as high as for analogue panoramic radiography.

1.6
Conventional Tomography

Because of the limitations of intra-oral or panoramic radiography with respect to bone quantity determination, other techniques are preferred which provide information on the bone volume in three dimensions. The principle of tomography is the simultaneous movement in opposite directions of the x-ray tube and the film. Movement can be linear or multidirectional.

For bone quantity assessment, cross-sectional tomographs of the bone are preferred. They are generally made on multidirectional tomographic equipment. Cross-sectional tomography implies an x-ray beam that is directed perpendicular to the bone curvature. Optimally, the tomographic plane should be at a right angle to the cortical border of the bone. Therefore, the tomographic plane should be individually selected for different areas of the horseshoe-shaped jaw. The latter may cause practical problems with regard to patient repositioning. In most of the linear tomographic equipments, the fulcrum of the moving parts of the radiographic equipment and the resulting magnification factors are variable. When the fulcrum is fixed, the magnification factor is also fixed. The problem of the magnification factor can partly be solved by introducing manual or computerised correction factors. This is needed for accurate bone height and bone width assessment.

Another problem is the rather limited resolution. Objects out of the tomographic layer are blurred, which may cause spurious contours. Measurements such as those of the cortical thickness are uncertain. The number of slices and the diagnostic value of the slices are restricted (Fig. 1.9). The exact localisation of the slices and the comparison with the conventional radiography are unclear. Inspection of the bone and identification of the anatomic structures are often not easy (Todd et al. 1993). Dental splints (stents) with radiopaque (metal) markers may be used as an aid to cross-sectional tomography. The radiopaque markers are placed in a hole drilled in the splint over the potential implant site. The splint is placed in the mouth before making the radiograph (Ismail et al. 1995). On cross-sectional images the markers are viewed in orovestibular and vertical dimension. On panoramic radiographs the markers are shown in a mesiodistal dimension. Due to image blurring and magnification, the technique

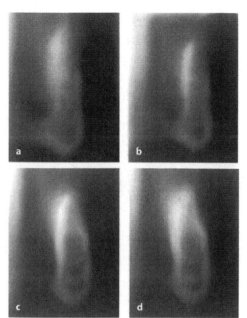

Fig. 1.9. A limited number of tomograms of an edentulous lower jaw are provided without clear indication of the scanned locations. Image blurring occurs and the mandibular canal is not well-defined. These drawbacks make interpretation of the tomograms difficult (from the Department of Radiology, University Hospital Gasthuisberg, Leuven, Belgium)

is of less interest and most often, computer tomography is preferred. Tomographs remain however a good alternative to reformatted CT scans when only limited information and detail of anatomic factors are needed.

A special multimodal radiographic equipment with a tomographic mode (Scanora, Soredex, Orion Corporation Ltd, Helsinki, Finland)(slice thickness 4mm) was found to give a better image quality than the conventional tomography (Ekestubbe and Gröndahl 1993). This multimodal radiography system utilises the principles of narrow beam radiography and spiral tomography (Fig. 1.10). While narrow beam radiography can be applied for detection of small jaw bone lesions, the spiral tomographic option (eight-turn spiral movement) can be applied for pre-operative planning of endosseous implants. One should take into account that this method has a constant magnification factor of 1.7 (Tammisalo et al. 1992; Ekestubbe and Gröndahl 1993). When using the Scanora system for planning implant placement, it is recommended to obtain first a panoramic radiograph to establish the co-ordinates of the area to be examined. Once these co-ordinates are determined, three or four tomograms are made during each imaging cycle. It should be emphasised that imaging by means of this technique will result in an effective dose equal to the panoramic image plus three to four times the dose reported for a single tomogram. Consequently the absorbed doses with the Scanora technique are higher than in the classical hypocycloidal tomography. For the maxilla, the dose is twice as high and for the mandible, 1,5 times (Ekestubbe et al. 1992). Furthermore, the effective dose delivered during multiple tomographic cuts needed for imaging of an entire maxillary bone is higher than for a reformatted CT scan examination (Kassebaum et al. 1992).

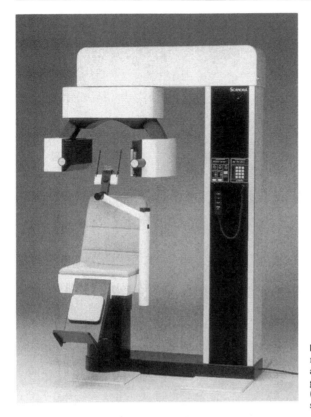

Fig. 1.10. This multimodal radiographic equipment enables both narrow beam radiography and spiral tomography (Courtesy from Soredex, Helsinki, Finland)

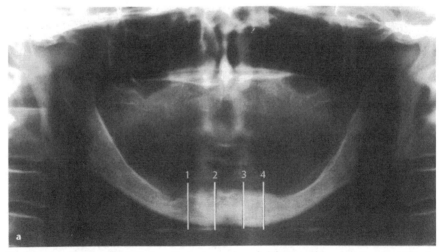

Fig. 1.11. Pre-operative planning of a patient, who needs a rehabilitation of the edentulous mandible. In this case, the Scanora equipment is used. After taking a panoramic radiograph (**a**), tomograms are made following the 4 lines indicated on the panoramic radiograph. Here only the tomogram, taken at line 3, is presented (**b**);

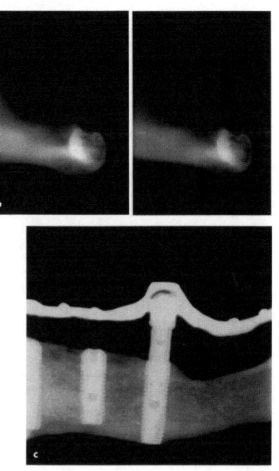

(Fig. 1.11)
The post-operative radiograph shows
three implants in the symphyseal area
(c) (Courtesy from Soredex, Helsinki,
Finland)

1.7
Computer Tomography (CT)

Computer tomography is the recommended imaging technique for implant treatment planning in the maxillae and distal areas of the mandible. It has been developed and clinically introduced by Hounsfield in the seventies. The technique is based on the principle of conventional tomography. The difference is that the radiograph is analogue-to-digitally converted to a computer image. Each point in the radiographic image has a certain density, which is dependent on the amount of absorbed radiation. By digital conversion, each point gets a grey value between 0 (black) and 255 (white), resulting in a matrix of picture elements, denoted as pixels. Computer-aided imaging allows manipulation and reconstruction of the data. It allows a far better visualisation of small density differences (by the technique of "window setting"). An important advantage for pre-operative planning is the significantly better visualisation of critical anatomic structures (e. g. the mandibular canal) when compared to conventional radiographs and tomographs. Pathological images like impacted roots, cysts or periodontal breakdown can be viewed in detail on the CT scan. CT scans not only provide information on the density values of cortical plates and medullar bone but can also be viewed three-dimensionally.

One should make a clear distinction between conventional (incremental) computer tomography and spiral CT. With conventional computer tomography, a thin cross-section of the human body or tomographic slice is examined from multiple angles using a narrowly collimated x-ray beam. The source (x-ray tube) and detectors are rigidly coupled and perform a rotational motion around the axis of the patient (1 slice). The transmitted radiation is counted by detectors and fed to a computer for further analysis. Conventional or incremental CT consists of successive scanning of single slices. The combined information of these slices inherently contains information about the three-dimensional anatomy of the imaged structure, although it is not visualised as such. Conventional CT scan analysis can be performed in different ways (Quirynen et al. 1990). In first, the direct technique includes coronal imaging in the lateral regions and sagittal imaging in the frontal region (Fig. 1.12). For screening of the whole jaw bone, 10 sagittal and 10 frontal images are required (slice thickness 1 – 2 mm). This technique can however lead to an overestimation of the available bone, especially in the canine/premolar region and therefore it is only recommended for use when imaging edentulous molar or incisor regions.

Two reformatting techniques (1. standard; 2. multiplanar reconstruction and display) are based on a series of axial scans taken in parallel to the lower border of the mandible or the hard palate. About 15 – 20 images are needed for the whole jaw (increments of table position 1 mm, slice thickness 2 mm). A standard reconstruction transforms axial slices to cross-sectional images. Reformatting occurs on the basis of the first axial scan that demonstrates the full jaw contour. A curve is superposed by the radiologist on this scan and centralised onto the jaw bone curvature. The computer

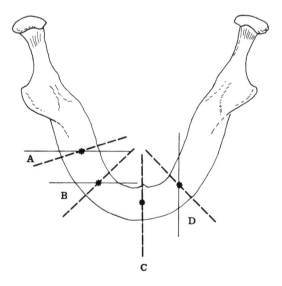

Fig. 1.12. Slice orientation in the molar (A), premolar (B), incisor (C) and canine (D) regions using direct coronal and sagittal images (solid line) and reconstruction techniques (dotted line). Applying the direct technique in the canine (D) or premolar (B) regions (solid lines) has the disadvantage of cutting through the neighbouring tooth regions as well. The bone height and bone width presented on the scan will thus provide a false impression of the actual bone present in the region to be examined (from Quirynen et al. 1990)

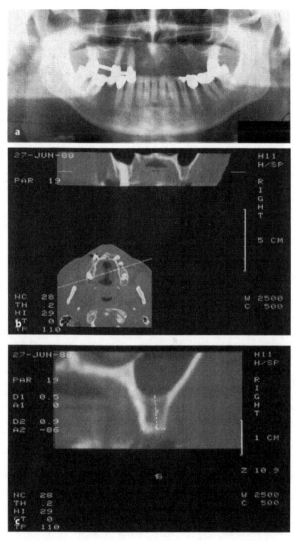

Fig. 1.13. Conventional CT-scan with standard reconstruction for pre-operative evaluation of an edentulous upper jaw. (a) Panoramic radiograph showing the edentulous regions in the upper jaw. (b) An axial scan at the level of the roots of the remaining teeth showing the position (line) of the reconstruction image. (c) The standard reconstruction in the region of the 16 demonstrate that there is enough bone below the maxillary sinus to place endosseous implants (from the Department of Radiology, University Hospital Gasthuisberg, Leuven, Belgium)

then generates a series of lines perpendicular to the previously drawn curve. These slices are numbered sequentially and can be varied from 1 to 10 mm apart (usually at 2-mm intervals). The numbers indicate the position of each axial slice and the corresponding cross-sectional image. In addition, the computer displays a ruler next to the image allowing measurements of the cross-sectional images. Multiplanar reconstructions are based on special reformatting-algorithms aiming to visualise the axial images in three dimensions. In the past, such a reformatting often resulted in geometrical errors and inaccurate assessment of the implant treatment planning. For the conventional CT-scan imaging, the standard reconstruction was therefore preferred as the technique for pre-operative planning (Quirynen et al. 1990)(Fig. 1.13).

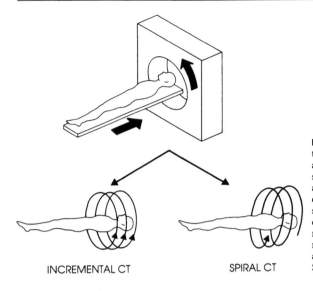

Fig. 1.14. With incremental CT, the x-ray source and detectors are rigidly coupled and perform several rotational movements around the patient, resulting in different individual slices. With spiral CT, the x-ray source and detectors perform one helical movement around the patient, resulting in continuous data acquisition (modified from Smet 1996)

Spiral CT (also denoted as "helical CT" or "volume-acquisition CT") is one of the latest technologies within CT imaging (Heiken et al. 1993). The patient undergoes a translation simultaneously with the rotation of the x-ray source ("spiral"), allowing a continuous information stream during scanning of the volume (Fig. 1.14). Image interpretation is analogous to that for conventional axial scanning. However, specific algorithms can be used to obtain reliable 2-D, 3-D and panoramic reconstruction. A 3-D presentation of the jaw bone has become possible. The axial plane is usually kept parallel to the palatum or the lower border of the mandible (slice thickness 1 mm). Spiral CT has a number of advantages as compared to incremental CT:

- reduced scanning time
- reduced radiation dose
- improved accuracy (slice thickness 0.4 to 1 mm)
- improved detection of small lesions
- improved 3-D reconstructions

In contrast to conventional cross-sectional tomography, CT reformatted images offer life size image presentation. A number of software packages have been developed for dental computer tomography :

- Dental CT (Siemens, Erlangen, Germany) allows multiplanar reformatting of data from the spiral CT, creating panoramic and 2-D cross-sectional images perpendicular on the jaw bone curvature
- Denta Scan (Dental Clinical Application Package, ISG Technologies, Inc., Missisaugua, Ontario, Canada) is another software package for panoramic and 2-D cross-sectional image formation of the mandible and maxilla
- Other software programs with similar scanning protocols include ToothPix (Cemax Inc., Fremont, Calif, USA) and 3-D Dental (Columbia Scientific Inc., Columbia, Md., USA)

These programs are specifically designed to avoid problems related to maxillofacial and oral imaging and creating more standardised images of the jaw bone: presence of metal artefacts (dental filling materials, prosthetic components), difficult positioning of the head (hyperflexion), reliability of the reformatted images. The use of dental splints with radiopaque markers can be recommended during the scanning procedure. These splints can be used to better orientate the possible implant site and axis. Based on the CT information, splints may also be used as a surgical guide during implant placement (see chapter 3).

The CT scan remains the most reliable and accurate imaging modality for pre-operative implant site assessment (Fig. 1.15). By further developments in computer tomography and optimisation of accompanying software programs, potential disadvantages such as the presence of "scatter artefacts" caused by dental metal restorations and the high radiation dosage for bone marrow, thyroid gland, salivary glands, eyes and skin (Fredholm et al. 1994), may be reduced in the future.

Depending on the extent of the jaw bone area to be investigated, it can be advantageous from a radiation exposure point of view to take either a spiral CT or only a few direct tomographic cuts. For a limited edentulous area it is evident that, unless there are stringent anatomic requirements, a few direct tomograms will give sufficient information. As stated before, one spiral CT of an edentulous jaw leads to less radia-

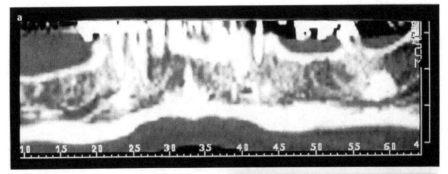

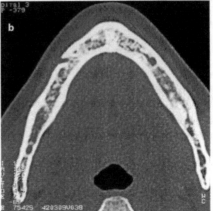

Fig. 1.15. Dental CT scan for pre-operative evaluation of a partially edentulous lower jaw in the left premolar and molar region. The panoramic radiograph indicates the location of the cross-sectional images by the numbers on the ruler (**a**). An axial scan showing the location of the mental foramen (**b**)

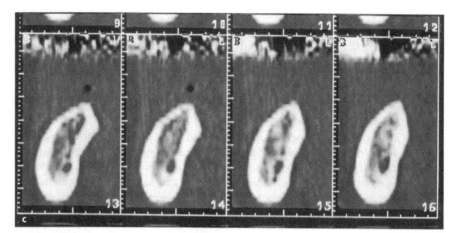

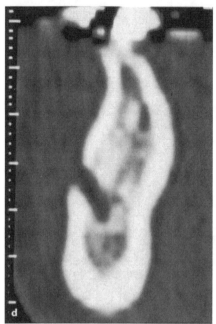

(Fig. 1.15)
Cross-sectional images in the molar **(c)** region
demonstrate that there is enough bone above the
canalis mandibularis to place endosseous
implants. A cross-sectional image through the
mental foramen helps to identify the location of
the canal on neighbouring slices **(d)** (from the
Department of Radiology, University Hospital
Gasthuisberg, Leuven, Belgium)

tion as compared to multiple conventional tomographic cuts. Following the radiological ALARA (as low as reasonably achievable) principle, it is justified to apply CT scan
imaging for pre-operative implant planning in the posterior mandible and in the
resorbed maxilla.

1.8
Recent Developments in Pre-Operative Treatment Planning

1.8.1
Interactive and Three-dimensional Computer Tomography

All the aforementioned imaging techniques are based on two-dimensional radiographs. Since the CT scan data contain information from the three dimensions, a three-dimensional presentation of the anatomic structures can be done but has not often been applied. One must realise that a surgeon works in a 3-D field while the radiographic information relating to the anatomic structures are provided in a 2-D mode. Thus, a mental transformation is required prior to and during surgery. Previous attempts to obtain a 3-D reconstruction by means of algorithms for multiplanar reformatting were often unreliable (geometrical errors). Recently, algorithmic transformations have been optimised to allow a better visualisation in the 3 dimensions. The main advantage of 3-D visualisations in diagnostics is that lesions can be seen from virtually any viewpoint (Grevers et al. 1991). It avoids the problem of mental reconstruction and allows easier, faster and improved analysis of complex structures (Bonnier et al. 1991; Luka et al. 1995). The most important therapeutic contribution of 3-D imaging is the facilitation of surgery planning (Luka et al. 1995). The extent of the surgery can be assessed, saving operative time and improving the post-operative result (Smet 1996). Shortcomings are the appearance of artefacts (motion, metal,...) and pseudoforamina, the absence of soft tissue visualisation, the loss of subtle surface detail and the increased time and effort (Ellis et al. 1992).

For pre-operative planning of oral implants, software programs are available to prepare and visualise the implant surgery interactively in 2-D (SimPlant, Columbia Scientific, Inc., Columbia, Maryland, USA). Attempts have also been made for planning of implant treatment with 3-D computer tomography (Jeffcoat 1992a). Recently, it became possible to visualise the anatomic structures in a 3-D mode on the computer screen for interactive implant placement on the computer (Verstreken et al. 1996)(Fig. 1.16). In the latter technique, even the reformatting from the original spiral CT data is performed on the workstation. First an individualised curvature is placed on one of the axial slices, after which the reformatting is analogous to that of the Dental CT software. The surgeon can interactively place implants on both the 2-D and 3-D computer images. The 2-D images are useful to take into account the bone anatomy and quality (thickness and location of the cortex), while the aesthetic and biomechanical adjustments (parallelism in between implants) can be carried out better from the 3-D image. Corrections in the 2-D images lead automatically to corrections in the 3-D images and vice-versa.

Further developments can lead to the combined use of 3-D reconstructions of CT slices and a computer-aided navigation system to allow maximal utilisation of local bone properties, accurate placement of implants and to avoid damage of neighbouring structures (Wagner et al. 1995).

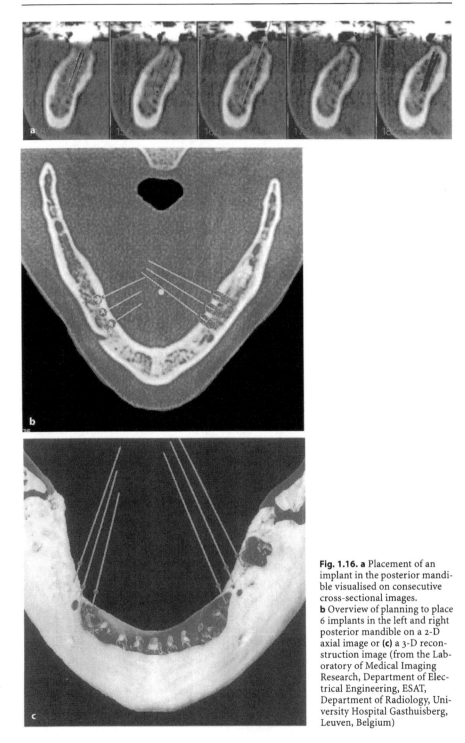

Fig. 1.16. a Placement of an implant in the posterior mandible visualised on consecutive cross-sectional images. **b** Overview of planning to place 6 implants in the left and right posterior mandible on a 2-D axial image or **(c)** a 3-D reconstruction image (from the Laboratory of Medical Imaging Research, Department of Electrical Engineering, ESAT, Department of Radiology, University Hospital Gasthuisberg, Leuven, Belgium)

1.8.2
Stereolithography

Stereolithography is a so-called Rapid Prototyping or Free Form Manufacturing procedure, which has an enormous growth potential within the biomedical sciences. Stereolithography can be applied in accurate modelling of different parts of the human body. The procedure of stereolithography is very similar to that of a CT scanner, where an anatomic region of the human body is sliced at regular intervals. Stereolithographic models are built up layer by layer. It is therefore quite obvious that the CT scan data can be applied for production of stereolithographic models. The distance between two subsequent images in a CT scan is usually 1 to 3 mm. For the stereolithographic process, this distance is reduced about 10 times, to meet the requirements regarding accuracy. A precision of less than 1 mm has been obtained for jaw models (Smet 1996). Anatomic models can be manufactured starting from standard CT scan data (Fig. 1.17). They can be used for visualisation of the real three-dimensional situation, for communication between clinicians and for demonstration to the patient. Stereolithographic models can be applied in complex maxillofacial surgery for visualisation, planning and implant design. One could also use the model for individualised modelling of an implant or a prosthesis, needed for the rehabilitation of a certain anatomic area. Actually, there are two techniques available for making the stereolithographic models (Lambrecht 1995). The first technique applies laser technology. An optical scanning system directs the laser which draws the image, one layer at the time onto a resin solution. As the laser strikes the surface, the resin is solidified and the first layer is built. This process is repeated and a second layer is built on top of the first. This continues until the entire model is built.

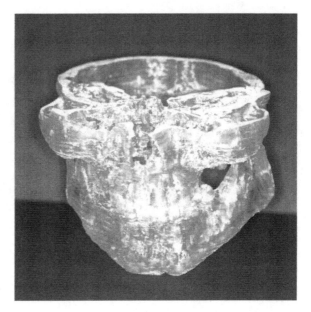

Fig. 1.17. Stereolithographic model based on data from the spiral CT (Courtesy from Materialise, Leuven, Belgium)

The second technique is based upon a computer-driven milling machine. Since the milling cutters work at high frequencies, they have a diameter of 2 – 6 mm in order to prevent instrumental deformation. The complexity of the jaw bone often requires a higher accuracy. As a consequence surface detail can be lost and hollow structures (e.g. mandibular canal) cannot be reproduced (Klein et al. 1992). Drawbacks of the stereolithographic technique in general are the limited accuracy, the need for an additional (3-D) CT – scan to visualise, manipulate and measure internal structures, the high costs and the limited availability of this technique. Therefore, stereolithography is restricted to complex surgery.

1.8.3
Magnetic Resonance Imaging (MRI)

In contrast to the aforementioned methods using x-rays for acquisition of information, the magnetic resonance technique applies non-ionising radiation. An MRI image is created by placing the patient in a large magnet, which induces a strong magnetic field. The nuclei of many atoms in the body align themselves with this magnetic field. When energy in the form of an electromagnetic wave is directed towards the tissue, energy will be absorbed by the tissue protons with a resonant frequency matching that of the electromagnetic wave. These protons will shift away from the direction induced by the imaging magnet. The absorbed energy is determined by the tissue characteristics and allows to differentiate between various anatomic structures. The resulting image is dependent on the strength of the magnetic field and the number of hydrogen nuclei present in the tissue.

This technique has two main advantages:

- the patient is not exposed to radiation since the technique is based on magnetism
- the soft tissue can be visualised

Based on hydrogen nuclei resonance, MRI is indeed particularly adapted to visualise water and lipids. Because of the soft tissue contrast obtained, it is useful in a variety of circumstances in the oral region:

- diagnosis of internal derangements of the temporo-mandibular joint (Hansson et al. 1992; De Laat et al. 1993) (Fig. 1.18)

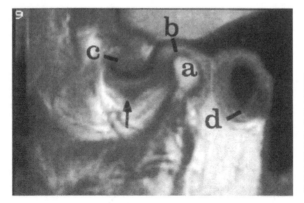

Fig. 1.18. Magnetic Resonance Image of the temporomandibular joint indicating anterior disc displacement (arrow) without reduction (closed lock): *a* processus condylaris, *b* fossa mandibularis, *c* tuberculum articulare, *d* meatus acousticus externus (from the Department of Radiology, University Hospital Gasthuisberg, Leuven, Belgium)

- identification and localisation of orofacial soft tissue lesions (Heffez et al. 1988)
- imaging of salivary gland parenchyma (Van den Akker 1988)

For visualising nonferromagnetic materials, MRI should be preferred to CT, where beam hardening artefacts usually degrade image quality severely. On the other hand, in patients with ferromagnetic metallic implants, MRI is contra-indicated because of the potential risks associated with movement or dislodgement of the objects (Shellock 1988). With regard to MRI of the maxillofacial region, non-precious ferromagnetic alloys (chrome-cobalt) produce large image deformations, whereas precious alloys (Au, Ag, Ti, amalgam) which are mainly non-ferromagnetic have no effect (Lissac et al. 1992). Other drawbacks are the high costs, long imaging time, critical patient collaboration (claustrophobia, movement artefacts). The latter implies that this technique is contra-indicated in young children. Considering the fact that MRI especially visualises the soft tissues, it should not yet be advocated for pre-operative planning of intra-oral implant placement.

1.9
Concluding Remarks

Considering the ALARA principle for pre-operative planning for implant placement, radiographic examination of the operation field is justified as the most important information source on the areas to be implanted. In selecting the most appropriate technique for pre-operative planning, it is needed to outweigh the effective dose of radiation (especially for radiosensitive tissues, see Table 1.3) against the required and also acquired information. One should take into account that a dose comparison for all techniques is influenced by the type, quality and quantity of the information obtained.

An important aspect in this discussion is the fact that implant surgery involves important investments (personnel, equipment, finance, stress) and normally occurs only once in a lifetime.

Table 1.3. Effective dose for intra-oral radiography, cephalography, panoramic radiography, conventional tomography, computer tomography (μSv) (modified from Frederiksen et al. 1994, 1995)

	intra-oral radiography*	panoramic radiography	tomography** anterior	premolar	molar	CT maxilla	CT mandible
Bone marrow	17	2	1	2	2	13	71
Oesophagus	1	3	1	4	4	14	34
Thyroid	47	4	1	5	5	19	72
Skin	1	<1	<1	1	<1	3	3
Bone surface	10	1	1	2	2	7	67
Salivary glands	–	16	2	17	13	45	510
Remainder	3	<1	<1	<1	<1	3	4
Sum	84	26	5	30	26	104***	761

* Intra-oral radiography is expressed as a full-mouth examination, being a series of 20 intra-oral radiographs (White 1992)
** Tomography is expressed as one slice. This means that if a full jaw must be visualised one should multiply these figures by at least 10
*** Low dose CT examinations lead to a further 40–65% decrease in the effective dose (Dula et al. 1996)

In Table 1.4 an attempt is made to indicate the technique of choice for a variety of indications.

Table 1.4. Advantages and disadvantages for each technique in pre-operative planning for implant placement

Imaging technique	Identification anatomic structures	Localisation anatomic structures	Image resolution	Image accuracy (real size?)	Total radiation risk relative to 1 intra-oral radiograph*	Accessibility	Costs	Indications for implant
intra-oral analogue	+	--	+	+	1	++	+	single tooth replacement
intra-oral digital	+/0	--	+/0	+	≤ 0.5	+	+	single tooth replacement
panoramic radiograph	0	+	-	-	6	++	+/0	symphyseal area mandible
lateral cephalogram	-	0	-	+	1**	+	0	implants + correction jaw relation
conventional tomogram	-	-	+	--	6-29 (per 4 tomograms)	-	-	1 or 2 implants; CT not available
spiral CT	++	++	++	++	25 (maxilla) 181 (mandible)	-	-	maxilla; lateral mandible
3-D CT	++	++	++	++	25 (maxilla) 181 (mandible)	--	--	maxilla; lateral mandible
stereolithography	+/0	++	0	-	25 (maxilla) 181 (mandible)	+	--	implants + complex surgery in maxillo-facial region
MRI	++	++	++	+	0	--	--	restricted to soft tissue lesions

Legends: -- negative; - relatively negative; o moderate; + good; ++ excellent for that criterion;
* values for expression of the total dose are derived from (White 1992; Frederiksen 1995)
** only with new cephalometric equipment having appropriate collimation

Chapter 2

Jaw Bone Quality and Quantity

2.1
Introduction

Prior to the actual pre-operative planning of implant placement, the restorative dentist and the periodontologist/oral surgeon should consider the patient's general health to establish whether there are any absolute or relative contra-indications for a surgical intervention and in particular the placement of implants. Psychiatric disorders, haemophilia and a recent myocardial infarction are typical examples of definite contra-indications. Diabetes, smoking, radiotherapy, sclerodermia are examples of relative contra-indications.

Once this is established, the radiographic techniques used to evaluate bone volumes in the areas considered for implantation should be carefully selected (see chapter 1). This examination should also include areas and structures other than the selected locations for implant installation (remaining teeth, sinuses) to evaluate whether there is any pathology which might interfere with the osseointegration process. It has indeed been documented that inflammatory foci in the immediate vicinity of implantation sites can interfere with bone apposition (van Steenberghe et al. 1990). Thus, the radiographic techniques applied should allow to detect the presence of inflammation of periodontal and endodontic origin and sinusitis, which need to be treated before the implant surgery is considered. The selected technique should also allow the clinician to detect and correctly locate any adjacent anatomic landmarks to be avoided, such as the mandibular canal and mental foramina, the nasal antrum and the maxillary sinus. These structures can be difficult to visualise especially in advanced resorption cases.

Since a limited bone volume leads to a less successful implant treatment outcome (van Steenberghe et al. 1990), the bone height expected to remain should be extrapolated from the radiographs taken prior to extraction (Atwood 1962). If deformities occur due to the imaging technique, the magnification factor must be known. Indeed, the surgeon must be able to check if the proper implant sizes are available with the manufacturer and if he has them in stock.

Determining the height of available bone is difficult. Indeed one should not opt for the maximally available distance, but take into account the inclination of the planned implant to meet the direction towards the occlusal plane it has to support. This is more or less set by the opposing teeth. Biomechanics is another factor that determines the inclination of the long axis of the implant and is mainly influenced by the presence of cortical plates. Thus one can deviate from the maximal length offered by a certain site of the jaw bone to meet other parameters from a biomechanical viewpoint. It is advisable that both the periodontologist/oral surgeon and the prosthodontist/restorative dentist evaluate simultaneously or consecutively the radiographs to optimise the chosen axis for implant placement. Networks will in the future allow us to look interactively from different sites to digital radiographs.

Besides the evaluation of bone quantity, jaw bone quality should also be taken into account. In contrast to a precise determination of absolute implant length, bone quality is usually assessed by a crude grading method. Whether such grading is sufficient for implant placement remains a matter of debate. It appears that radiographic and per-operative (during drilling) assessments of bone density seem to coincide rather well (Lekholm and Zarb 1985). It should be considered that bone quality has a strong influence on implant success (Jaffin and Berman 1991). Poor bone quality does not offer the necessary primary stability to allow optimal bone healing after insertion of an implant. It could also be argued that information on bone quality is required for an optimised biomechanical design of the prosthetic superstructure. Cutting resistance during implant insertion can be measured with a computerised equipment connected to the torque motor (Johansson and Strid 1994; Friberg et al. 1995).

2.2
The Mandible

A number of anatomic landmarks are important to consider during a pre-operative examination. The most important is the mandibular canal which contains a neurovascular bundle including the afferents from the incisor region and from the mental nerve. The latter is responsible for the tactile sensation of the homolateral lower lip. Any disturbance of this nerve or its afferents will lead to a lasting an-, hypo- or paraesthesia. Since edentulism of the lateral parts of the mandible must sometimes be rehabilitated by means of implants, evaluation of the bone above or besides the canal is often challenging. Lack of precision of a radiographic technique will lead to either a too cautious approach or to damage of the nerve. In the former case, the available bone volume is not optimally used, in the latter moral or even legal consequences result. In general, the mental nerve enters the mandible in the parasymphy-

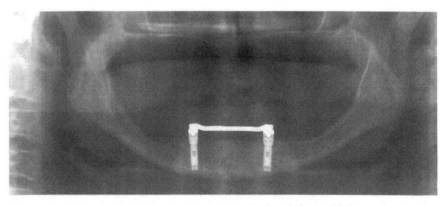

Fig. 2.1. Panoramic radiograph of a severely resorbed mandible with the mandibular canal on top of the jaw bone. Two implants have been installed in the symphyseal area

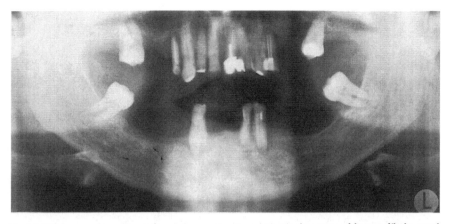

Fig. 2.2. This panoramic radiograph reveals an anatomic variation in the course of the mandibular canal with an anterior loop of the canal and the mental foramen almost on top of the mandibular bone (arrows). The latter has important consequences to determine the strategy of implant surgery

seal area which corresponds to the first and second premolar location in the presence of teeth. The bone resorption resulting from the loss of teeth leads to a decrease of the distance between the mental foramen and the bone crest. Sometimes the nerve can even lie on top of the bone (Fig. 2.1). When entering the foramen, the nerve often loops anteriorly in the incisive canal. It rapidly moves distally and progressively more lingually, having a slight curvature with a caudal convexity. The alveolar nerve bundle as it is called as soon as the mental nerve fuses with the incisive nerve, is further joined by more afferents throughout its course, before emerging at the lingual site of the ramus ascendens at the mandibular foramen. Since important individual variations occur, one cannot rely on the general course outline or extrapolate from one visible part to another, because the canal sometimes has a wavy anatomy (Nortje et al. 1977; Yosue and Brooks 1989 a+b). In Fig. 2.2, the panoramic radiograph of a partially edentulous patient reveals an anatomic variation of the course of the mandibular canal, having important consequences for the planning of implant surgery.

When the jaw bone is poorly mineralised, the increased bone density around the canal, some speak of a corticalisation, can be absent rendering the visualisation of the canal difficult (Fig. 2.3)

In the most distal parts of the corpus mandibulae, where implant installation is more and more considered in the perspective of providing anchorage to allow orthodontic tooth displacement, the thick cortex of the anterior border of the ramus ascendens and the linea obliqua externa, regularly mask the canal. The same applies to exostoses, which are localised protuberances on the surface of the bone and appear as areas of increased radiographic density.

As resorption of the lower jaw bone progresses, the intermaxillary relationship changes in a frontal plane. Besides, an increasing concavity develops at the lingual side of the corpus mandibulae. The thinning of the remaining alveolar process means that regularly the bone height measured on the two-dimensional radiographic

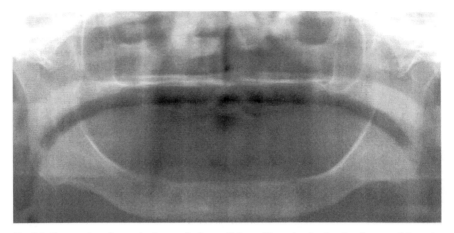

Fig. 2.3. Panoramic radiograph of a resorbed mandible unable to clearly visualise the mental foramina and mandibular canal

images is of insufficient width to harbour an implant. Because of the pronounced inclination of the mandibular bone in a lingual direction, this should be duly recognised to avoid any risk of perforating the lingual cortex during drilling procedures. Indeed, the intimate relationship between the mylohyoid artery and the horizontal mandibular body implies the risk of a serious bleeding difficult to control since the artery runs caudal to the mylohoid muscle. All these arguments should urge the clinicians to opt for the most precise radiographic technique available, taking into account the liabilities of the radiation involved. One should strongly oppose the tradition of some dentists to prefer chairside radiology in contrast with the rest of medicine. Indeed, the radiographic examination for planning implant placement is not urgent. Since it is a more or less unique event in a patient's life, one should not be refrained from the optimal technique.

There have been numerous studies to compare the merits of different radiographic techniques in evaluating the height of the bone above the canal (Wical and Swoope 1974; Van Waas 1983). Several comparative studies indicate that both the exactness of location and the frequency of visualisation of the mandibular canal are superior with a reformatted CT scan technique than with other techniques, including tomographic examinations (Klinge et al. 1989; Lindh et al. 1992; Sonick et al. 1994; Fritz 1996)(Table 2.1). As stated on the World Workshop in Periodontics 1996, reformatted CT scans "... allow the use of maximal available bone height and enable the clinician to discover pre-operatively if sufficient bone volume is available in the maxilla and the mandible" (World Workshop in Periodontics 1996).

By using data from CT scans, the clinician can circumvent the canal on either buccal or lingual side, if adequate bone exists in these areas. In Fig. 2.4 the visibility of the mandibular canal on CT scans is illustrated in one partially edentulous patient. The radiographic examination of the anterior mandible, i.e. in between the mental foramina is less demanding. Indeed, there are no anatomic structures to be avoided. Damaging the remains of the involuted incisive nerves does not lead to sensory disturbances. If a radiopaque standard is placed intra-orally, one can calculate the bone

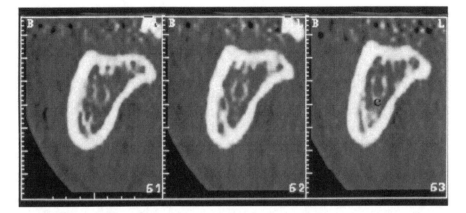

Fig. 2.4. Cross-sectional images of a spiral CT scan illustrate the visibility of the mandibular canal (c) (from the Department of Radiology, University Hospital Gasthuisberg, Leuven, Belgium)

height with relatively good precision on a simple panoramic radiograph. One can simply determine the magnification factor in different areas using standards with a known length and diameter. The real bone height can then be calculated as the ratio between the measured bone height and the magnification factor (Table 2.2).

The latter will however not reveal the bone width or the extent of lingual concavities especially encountered in the very resorbed lower jaw. Indeed, the fossa sublingualis can be challenging during drilling procedures in that area. The same applies to the appearance of an anterior buccal mandibular depression, which is more readily detected on CT scans than on panoramic radiographs (Littner et al. 1995). The use of a lateral cephalogram will not be helpful, since it only reveals the bone volume at the midline, while the concavities mentioned are paramedian. A cephalogram gives an overestimation of both quantitative and qualitative bone parameters of the symphyseal area and cannot be recommended when planning oral implant placement. With

Table 2.1. Accuracy to locate the mandibular canal using different imaging techniques (modified from Klinge et al. 1989, Sonick et al. 1994)

radiographic technique	% of measurements within 1 mm of true value	distortion average in mm	average in %	range in %
intra-oral	53	1.9	14.0	8–24
panoramic	17	3.0	23.5	5–39
CT scan	91	0.2	1.8	0–9

Table 2.2. Equations for bone height calculations from magnified radiographs

$$\text{magnification factor} = \frac{\text{measured dimensions standard}}{\text{real dimensions standard}}$$

$$\text{real bone height} = \frac{\text{measured bone height}}{\text{magnification factor}}$$

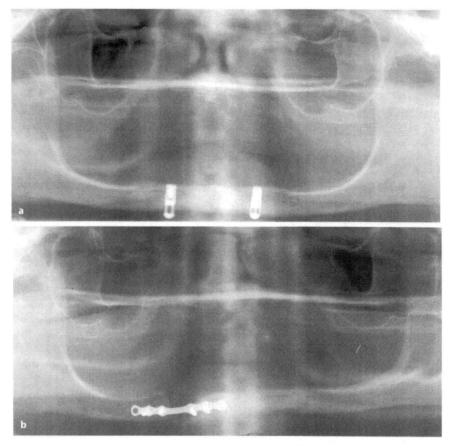

Fig. 2.5. Panoramic radiograph showing a severely resorbed mandible. Implants had to be removed because of non-osseointegration **(a)**. This led to a fracture of the mandible **(b)**. In such a case, additional information on the bone width might be required (CT scanning), to estimate the fracture risk

extreme bone resorption, a CT examination with reformatting can be useful for assessment of fracture risk after implant placement (Fig. 2.5). Also, when the anterior mandible is very thin, a marked radiolucency may occur in the incisive region on the panoramic radiograph even if hardly any medullary space is present. Although this is not a pathologic condition, additional information on the width of the mandibular symphyseal bone is required to evaluate if it is safe for implant placement.

While the jaw bone has been traditionally evaluated using panoramic and intra-oral films, CT scanning has provided a new look at the mandible and the maxilla (Abrahams 1993). When evaluation data gathered with the Dental CT software, cross-sectional, axial and panoramic views are provided, giving detailed information on the anatomic structures in the 3 dimensions (Fig. 2.6).

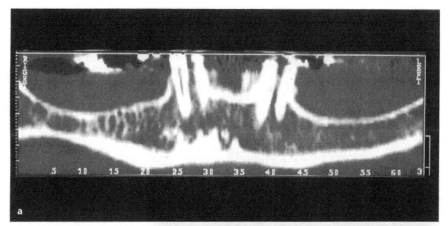

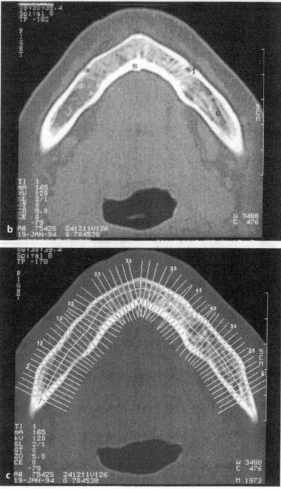

Fig. 2.6. Panoramic views indicate the inferior mandibular canal, the mental foramen, the amount of cortical and trabecular bone **(a)**. Axial views may illustrate the inferior mandibular canal (c), the mental foramen (f) and the mental spines (s) **(b)**. Cross-sectional views are reformatted along the numbered lines on the axial view **(c)** and the corresponding numbers on the panoramic view **(a)**

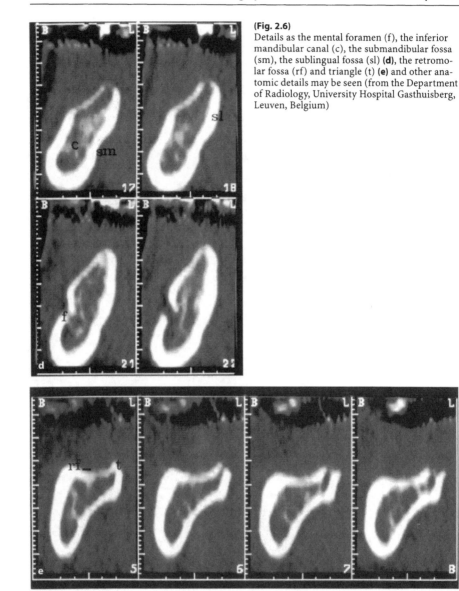

(Fig. 2.6)
Details as the mental foramen (f), the inferior mandibular canal (c), the submandibular fossa (sm), the sublingual fossa (sl) **(d)**, the retromolar fossa (rf) and triangle (t) **(e)** and other anatomic details may be seen (from the Department of Radiology, University Hospital Gasthuisberg, Leuven, Belgium)

2.3
The Maxilla

In the maxilla, after extraction of teeth, bone resorption may progress to the extent that only a thin layer of bone remains to cover the floor of the maxillary sinus and the nasal fossae. The bone itself can also become thin in a labio-oral plane throughout the maxilla.

The incisive foramen (anterior palatine foramen) on the oral side of the nasopalatine canal transmits terminations of the greater palatine artery and of the nasopalatine nerve (which participates in the innervation of the maxillary incisors and surrounding structures). The anterior palatine foramen is situated in the anterior portion of the midline of the palate. Its radiographic appearance varies markedly in shape, size, and sharpness. Its image varies in relation to the roots of the incisor teeth, and ranges from a position near the alveolar bone level to one at the level of the apex of the roots. It may be superimposed on the apex of the central incisor and mistaken for a periapical lesion. It may also be confused with a cyst of the incisive canal, which has a well-defined border and tends to be round. The presence of a cyst is presumed when the width of the foramen exceeds 10 mm (Fig. 2.7).

During pre-surgical implant assessment, one has to take into account the width of the foramen, which varies greatly. The anterior palatine or nasopalatine canal is not always visualised through radiographs such as panoramic or even intra-oral radiographs (Fig 2.8). It can be perceived as two radiopaque lines, one extending downward from the floor of each nasal fossa. The fatty tissue within the canal can contaminate the implant surface during insertion and thus interfere with bone apposition, which is an essential aspect of osseointegration. This probably explains the higher failure rates of implants placed in the immediate vicinity of the canal. The nasopalatine canal originates from two foramina in the floor of the nasal cavity. The superior foraminae of the incisive canal are often visualised on radiographs of the maxillary lateral incisors and canines. They appear as round or oval radiolucent areas in the floor of the nasal fossae and near the nasal septum. On reformatted CT scans the incisive canal is always well visible. The same applies to other anatomic structures (Fig. 2.9).

Maxillary sinuses vary greatly in size, some being so small that evidence of them does not appear on an intra-oral radiograph. Others are so large because they extend downward after tooth extraction. The size may also vary from one side to another in the same patient. The evaluation of the bone volume present below the maxillary sinuses can only be properly carried out through CT examinations with reformatted images (Andersson and Kurol 1987; Andersson and Svartz 1988; Duckmanton et al. 1994). Especially in situations with reduced bone height (<15 mm), in which oral implants are sometimes needed, CT images provide more accurate information during pre-operative planning (Lam et al. 1995). If not, now and then, one will find that after reflecting the mucoperiosteum, the surgery has to be interrupted because of an insufficient bone volume.

Prior to implant placement, it is also important to diagnose the presence of maxillary sinusitis. Indeed, inflammatory reactions in the vicinity of an implantation site are unfavourable for the bone apposition process. Acute sinusitis is recognised by a uniform cloudiness or abnormal increased radiopacity of the sinus (Schwarz et al. 1989). Chronic sinusitis is recognised by irregular areas of density which are evidence of an uneven sclerosing of the antral bone and thickened antral mucosa and perhaps the presence of polyps. During a pre-operative examination, the patient has to be informed about the diagnosis of sinusitis, to avoid post-operative complaints of the patient who might relate the occurrence of sinusitis to the implant installation. The same applies to roots and foreign bodies in the sinus. Foreign bodies may be introduced through a bucco-sinusal opening during dental treatment and when they are

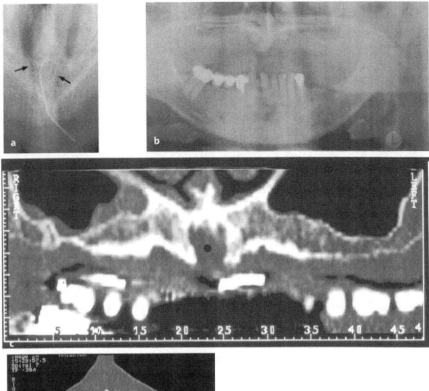

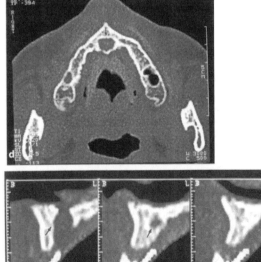

Fig. 2.7. Intra-oral radiograph of the maxillary incisor region, showing the appearance of an enlarged nasopalatine canal (arrow). The gutta percha point was inserted to visualise the fistula **(a)**. The panoramic radiograph does not reveal a clear radiolucency **(b)**, whereas the panoramic view of the CT scan indicates the presence of a nasopalatine cyst **(c)**(ball). This is also visualised by the axial **(d)** and cross-sectional **(e)** views of the CT scan (arrow) (from the Department of Radiology, University Hospital Gasthuisberg, Leuven, Belgium)

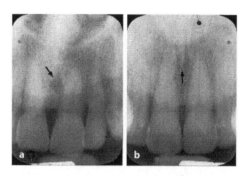

Fig. 2.8. Appearance on an intra-oral radiograph of the: **a** incisive foramen (arrow), **b** nasopalatine canal (arrow)

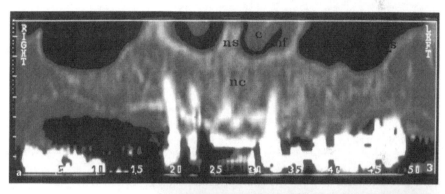

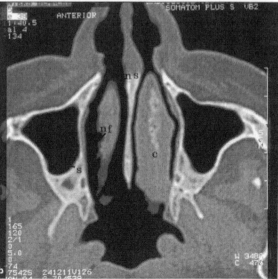

Fig. 2.9. The Dental CT software offers panoramic views which reveal the nasopalatine canal (nc), the nasal fossae (nf), conchae (c) and nasal septum (ns) together with the maxillary sinuses (s) **(a)**. On the axial image, the same structures can be identified with more sharpness (not reformatted) **(b)**

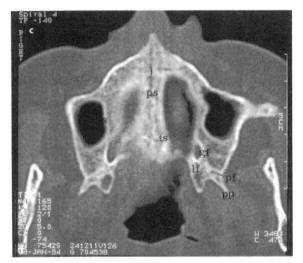

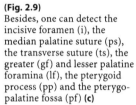

(Fig. 2.9)
Besides, one can detect the
incisive foramen (i), the
median palatine suture (ps),
the transverse suture (ts), the
greater (gf) and lesser palatine
foramina (lf), the pterygoid
process (pp) and the pterygo-
palatine fossa (pf) **(c)**

radiopaque they can be identified on an intra-oral radiograph. Other abnormalities of the sinus are less frequent but have to be considered prior to implant installation. An odontogenic cyst for example, is manifested as a round uniform radiolucency bordered by a thin, radiopaque margin. A mucoid retention cyst has its origin in the sinusal mucosa. It is recognised on a radiograph by its radiopaque, dome-shaped or hemispherical form, with the antral wall as base. Tumours originate in the sinus or involve secondarily the sinus. Any radiographic destruction of the antral wall should be suspected as being caused by a tumour.

In full edentulism, it seems sufficient to install 4 to 6 implants in between the maxillary sinuses to support afterwards a full bridge up to the first molar area. The number of implants that can be installed in between the sinuses can best be determined on axial slices of the CT scan. Long-term data of one implant system indicates that even after 10 years of observation there is no significant difference in success rate between bridges on 4 or 6 implants (Brånemark et al. 1995). The clinician should thus carefully calculate how much space is available and not try to squeeze in too many implants.

Often patients and even clinicians think there is a need to rehabilitate the entire dental arch in full edentulism. There is ample evidence from the dentate situation that a symmetrical rehabilitation up to the second or first premolar respectively for patient groups below and above 45 years of age meets all functional and subjective requirements (Witter et al. 1989). One should not try to insert implants in the lateral regions of the maxilla in full edentulism when not needed and certainly refrain from systematic sinus inlay grafting which seems to be fashionable in some centres nowadays. This is rather implantology and not oral rehabilitation by means of implants.

The axial slices of the CT scan allow the surgeon to plan the placement of implants in the most archwise configuration as possible. This means that the distal implants are preferrably placed in an oral position and the anterior ones rather labially. Indeed

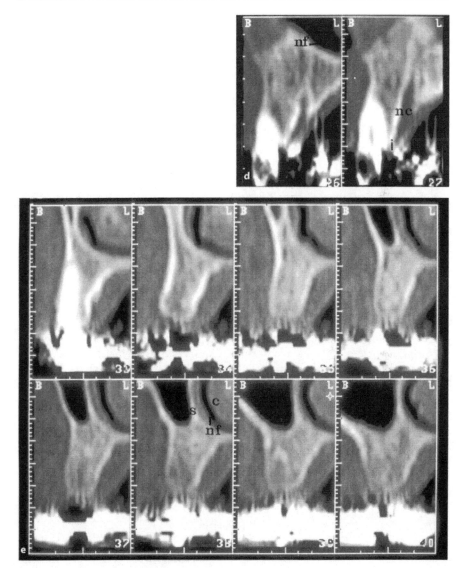

(Fig. 2.9) The cross-sectional views also reveal the cortical plate **(d, e)** (from the Department of Radiology, University Hospital Gasthuisberg, Leuven, Belgium)

from a biomechanical point of view, when distal cantilevers are needed in a fully edentulous jaw, the implants should not be installed along one axis which would result in important cantilever forces (Rangert 1993).

The axial slices will help the prosthodontist or restorative dentist to fabricate a template. This template can be used by the surgeon to find the proper locations for the placement of implants. A wide nasopalatine canal may prevent implant placement in central incisor locations. If sufficient mesiodistal space is available, one will choose implant sites in the more lateral areas giving more freedom for the restoration of the central incisors as well as helping to achieve better aesthetics.

The CT-reformatted image will also allow an evaluation of the bone volume available in the tuberosity regions. When the maxillary sinuses have expanded, especially in a mesial direction, there can be a need to establish support for the dental prosthesis in the distal areas. When for example the most available distal maxillary location in the frontal part is the canine area, the cantilever might be too long even when the implants can be placed in an archwise fashion.

Three alternatives with sufficient documentation then exist:

- an overdenture or removable metallic prosthesis on a rigid bar on 4 implants
- the placement of implants distal to the maxillary sinus
- the placement of autologous bone graft in the sinus in conjunction with or followed by implants

The study of the CT scan data from the tuberosity region will influence the final choice between these options.

It should also be stressed that implant placement in the maxilla may be compromised by poor quality bone. Fine bony detail is not always apparent on conventional tomography, but can be reliably assessed on computer tomography (Schwarz et al. 1989; Duckmanton et al. 1994).

In conclusion, it could be stated that CT-scanning of the maxilla provides comprehensive information of relevant bony structures, bone quality and soft tissues. Using CT-scans, the width of the paranasal sinuses, nasal cavity and incisive canal can be properly evaluated. The measurements of available space on the CT images will allow a precise determination of the positions, inclinations, number and lengths of implants to be installed.

Chapter 3

Radiographic Indications and Contra-Indications for Implant Placement

3.1
Introduction

Prior to placement of implants, a routine oral examination should be carried out. All information needed for the treatment planning should be gathered. Radiographic information should include a complete röntgen-status using the long-cone paralleling technique or – when only few teeth are present – a combination of a panoramic radiograph and a selected number of intra-oral radiographs.

It is important to determine that the bone has the necessary quantity and quality to provide a sufficient support for the implant. Lekholm and Zarb (1985) introduced a simple grading system for rapid assessment of bone quality and quantity on pre-operative radiographs (panoramic, CT) and/or during surgery. Jaw bone quality is assessed on the basis of the amount of cortical bone and the morphology of the trabecular bone. Better bone quality is obtained with greater thickness of cortical bone (grade 1 and 2). Less cortical bone (grade 3) combined with thinner cancellous bone and larger trabecular spaces (grade 4) offers less favourable implant support. Bone quantity is assessed according to the morphology of the edentulous mandible or maxilla varying from grade A (most of alveolar ridge present) to grade E (extreme resorption of the basal bone).

A patient being screened for endosseous implants should have a minimum radiographic examination consisting of intra-oral radiographs and/or panoramic radiographs. Reformatted CT scans should supplement the screening examination when jaw bone dimensions and anatomic limitations are challenging. The accuracy and resolution of reformatted CT scans are superior to other radiographic imaging tech-

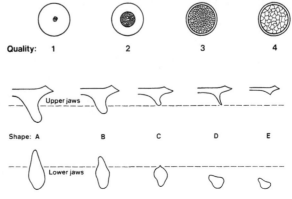

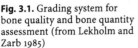

Fig. 3.1. Grading system for bone quality and bone quantity assessment (from Lekholm and Zarb 1985)

niques to identify anatomic landmarks such as the mandibular canal. It allows the use of maximal available bone height and enables the clinician to discover preoperatively if sufficient bone volume is available in the maxilla and the mandible.

Although the total radiation dose of CT scans is higher than that of conventional tomography, it does not involve the more radiosensitive tissues in the adjacent areas (thyroid, pituitary gland) and presents an acceptable radiation risk. Tomographs might be an alternative to reformatted CT scans when limited detail of anatomic factors are needed. For the different imaging techniques applied, radiopaque templates allow a more precise localisation of potential implant sites and may serve as a surgical guide to optimise prosthetics (see § 3.4).

3.2
Radiographic Indications

3.2.1
Full edentulism

Edentulism creates physiologic and psychological problems. Reduced stability and retention of the dentures, especially in the mandible lead to a compromised functional capacity. Both overdentures on two implants connected with a bar and four to six implants supporting a full fixed prostheses have been advocated to solve those problems (Figs. 3.2, 3.3).

Whether to choose the one or the other solution depends on the economic, psy-

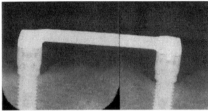

Fig. 3.2. Edentulous patient rehabilitated with an overdenture on two implants connected with a bar in the lower jaw

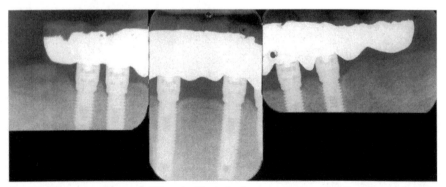

Fig. 3.3. Edentulous patient rehabilitated with six implants supporting a full fixed prosthesis in the lower jaw

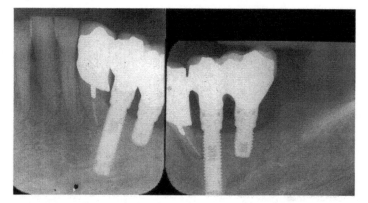

Fig. 3.4. Periodontitis was not treated prior to implant installation which is detrimental for the osseointegration

chological, aesthetic and functional factors. It has been demonstrated that the majority of elderly patients are more satisfied with an overdenture on implants (Feine et al. 1994 a, b). On the other hand, one must also consider the ongoing bone resorption in the posterior mandible and the maxillary front region. The latter tends to be increased when opposing a full fixed prosthesis in the lower jaw (Jacobs et al. 1992; 1993). When the patient asks for a rehabilitation of both upper and lower jaws and the requirements of jaw bone quantity and quality are fulfilled, a full fixed prosthesis in both upper and lower jaws can be considered. Besides rehabilitation with full fixed prostheses, one could also opt for overdenture on 2 interconnected implants in the lower jaw or 4 implants connected by a bar in the upper jaw. Indeed, in the upper jaw an overdenture on 2 implants has been associated with important marginal bone loss and high failure rates (Quirynen et al. 1991a).

3.2.2
Partial Edentulism

Implant treatment of partially edentulous patients differs in many ways from that of the edentulous ones. Multi-centre observations however indicate that good results can be obtained with a 5-years observation span (Lekholm et al. 1994). In analogy with the completely edentulous subjects, implants fail more often when a reduced bone quantity and quality is present. In partial edentulism, it is essential to treat periodontal inflammatory conditions first to reduce the incidence of failures (van Steenberghe et al. 1990)(Fig. 3.4).

3.2.3
Single Tooth Replacement

Implants can be successfully installed at the time of tooth extraction or after either soft or hard tissue healing (Tolman and Keller 1991; Laney et al. 1994). In a number of these cases, the use of autografts, allografts or e-PTFE membranes has been advocated (Wilson 1992; Simion et al. 1994; Becker et al. 1994).

3.2.4
Extreme Jaw Bone Resorption in the Mandible

As long as 6 mm bone height and 5 mm vestibulo-oral bone width is available, endos-seous implants can be placed. Such a severely resorbed mandible may present a frac-ture risk during implant placement (Laney and Tolman 1989). However, the need for implant rehabilitation in such a patient is often higher than in the others. One should therefore carefully consider the individual patient. There is a dilemma between an increased fracture risk when installing 4 to 6 implants for a fixed prosthesis and an increased risk for nerve compression or irritation of the mental nerve on top of the mandible when installing 2 implants connected by a bar to retain an overdenture. Another drawback of this resilient design is the ongoing bone resorption in the poste-rior mandible (Jacobs et al. 1992).

3.2.5
Extreme Jaw Bone Resorption in the Maxilla

In the upper jaw , the minimal bone volume needed is a 7 mm bone height and 4 mm vestibulo-oral bone width. To support a full fixed prosthesis in the upper jaw, 4 to 6 implants may be installed in between the maxillary sinuses with a similar success rate (Brånemark et al. 1995). Even with 7 mm implants acceptable results have been obtained.

3.3
Radiographic Contra-Indications

Radiographic contra-indications include those situations in which implant place-ment is compromised by local or systemic bone factors. In most instances, treatment can deal with these factors. As stated before, it is possible to treat virtually all patients. On the other hand, psychiatric disorders, some coagulation disorders and a recent myocardial infarction may be strong contra-indications. Diabetes, smoking, radio-therapy, sclerodermia only seem relative contra-indications.

3.3.1
Severely Resorbed Jaw Bone

If less than 6 mm bone height and 5 mm bone width is available in the mandible, an onlay autologous bone graft can be considered (van Steenberghe et al. 1991) (Fig. 3.5a). In the upper jaw, the minimal bone volume needed is 7 mm bone height and 4 mm vestibulo-oral bone width. When less bone is available, one may consider to install fewer implants (on these locations with enough bone) or to opt to increase the bone volume by means of an autologous iliac crest bone graft (Triplett and Schow 1996) (Fig. 3.5b).

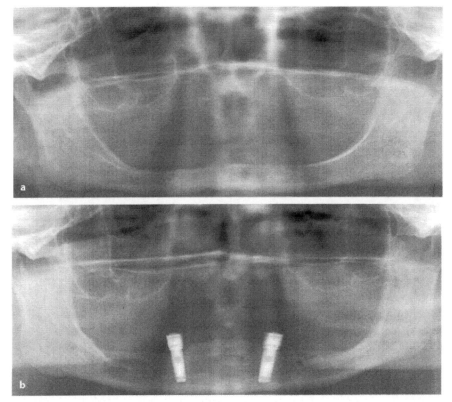

Fig. 3.5. Panoramic radiography of a severely resorbed jaw bone **(a)**, indicating the use of an autologous bone graft and 2 osseointegrated implants to rehabilitate the mandible **(b)**

3.3.2
Systemic Diseases

The intra-oral radiograph often provides information that is valuable in the identification and diagnosis of a systemic disease. In some instances, it may even be the first clue leading to an early diagnosis of the disease. Prior to implant treatment, a correct diagnosis and treatment of these diseases is essential. In general, every radiograph showing an abnormal bone pattern has to be considered thoroughly taking the clinical symptoms and medical history into account, to exclude systemic diseases prior to implant installation. Common metabolic bone disorders such as renal osteodystrophy, osteomalacia and Paget's disease could compromise bone remodelling after implant installation (Roberts et al. 1992). The most prevalent problem however is osteoporosis. Unfortunately, oral radiography cannot be applied to identify osteoporosis in an individual patient (von Wowern and Kollerup 1992). Furthermore, osteoporosis only plays an important role once teeth have been extracted. In partially edentulous subjects, local factors play the primary role in bone remodelling. According to Dao and co-workers (1993), osteoporosis seems not to be a risk factor for rehabilitation with implants.

3.3.3
Congenital Defects

In a number of congenital defects, rehabilitation by means of implants may be the treatment modality of choice. However, a multidisciplinary approach and thorough pre-operative planning is required. When teeth are missing such as in hypodontia or oligodontia, there is an associated failure of normal development of the corresponding portion of the alveolar process, which may result in an inadequate width for implant placement. For complete anodontia, autogenous bone grafting in conjunction with implant placement is often required. Edentulous patients with persistent cleft palate defects may be provided with a bone-anchored prosthesis, replacing teeth and obturating the oronasal communication. When the available bone volume is inadequate, autogenous bone grafting may also be needed. For rehabilitation of craniofacial defects, pre-operative planning is much more complex. It requires additional radiographic examination, preferably by using 3-D CT images or stereolithography.

3.3.4
Irradiation

Irradiated bone has a lowered vitality and in some instances osteoradionecrosis occurs. This may be identified by increased radiographic density, followed by evidence of osteolytic centres. Following irradiation, surgical intervention should be avoided, but irradiated patients are often the most needy ones. It seems that with a long enough recovery period after irradiation, treatment with implants and facial or dental prostheses is successful (Taylor and Worthington 1993). Marx and Johnson (1987) rather advocate surgery as soon as possible after irradiation. To reduce the risk for osteoradionecrosis, one may attempt to revitalise irradiated bone by means of a hyperbaric oxygen therapy prior to implant surgery (Myers and Marx 1990; Granström 1992).

3.3.5
Infection

Intra-oral radiographs provide a detailed image of the remaining teeth and their periodontal condition. This kind of images also give information on the quality of dental care. Caries lesions and peri-apical infections must be eliminated prior to implant surgery. Periodontal breakdown identified on a intra-oral radiograph may be an indication of sensitivity to periodontitis, but the relationship with peri-implantitis is not established. Implant loading seems to be more important than plaque with regard to implant failure in two-stage implants (Quirynen et al. 1992c). In a long-term perspective the presence of gingivitis seems to be associated with increased marginal bone loss (Lindquist et al. 1996). Still, periodontitis should be treated prior to implant placement for several reasons: surgery and healing in an "healthy" environment, treatment planning and individual prognosis of teeth, patient motivation, ... (Fig. 3.6a) (van Steenberghe et al. 1990). Retained roots in the jaw bone should be detected and removed, since they may interfere with implant installation (infection and

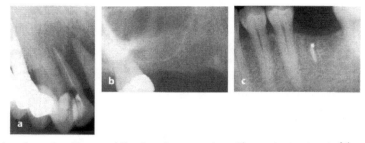

Fig. 3.6. Implants have been placed in a partially edentulous upper jaw without prior treatment of the periodontal infection (**a**). Prior to implant placement a root remnant (**b**) or a foreign body (**c**) should be removed

implant failure) (Fig. 3.6b). Localised areas of compact sclerotic bone (condensing osteitis / osteosclerosis) may form obstacles for implant installation.

3.3.6
Cysts, Tumours and Fibro-Osseous Lesions of the Jaw Bone

Epithelium-lined cysts appear radiographically as fairly uniform radiolucent cavities in the bone, with a well-defined circumscribed border. The identification and elimination of these cysts prior to implant surgery, is essential (Fig. 3.7). The same applies to odontogenic tumours. Their radiographic appearance depends on the nature, location and stage of development. A radiograph is also very important in revealing the presence of non-odontogenic tumours in the jaw bone. Benign tumours tend to be demarcated from the surrounding bone by well-defined margins, while the cortex remains intact. In contrast, the malignant tumour often involves destruction of the cortex and has irregular borders fading into the surrounding bone.

3.3.7
Foreign Bodies

Foreign bodies in the soft tissue as well as those within the jaws are frequently encountered during routine intra-oral radiographic examination (Fig. 3.6c). By taking radiographs in different incidences combined with an occlusal radiograph, the location of foreign bodies in the soft tissue can be identified. Foreign bodies commonly found within the jaws are amalgam, gutta percha, cements and pieces of dental instruments. Nowadays, bone lesions are regularly filled with all kinds of implantable materials. One has to be sure that implants are not installed in bone defects filled with

Fig. 3.7. Peri-apical radiolucencies are visible around the roots of a premolar and a molar tooth (**a**). After extraction of these teeth with subsequent implant placement, an apical radiolucency is visible around the mesial implant (**b**). Eventually, this could be related to the presence of the chronic infection

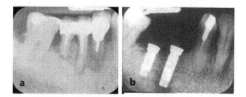

these kinds of materials. They may interfere with the osseointegration process and increase the post-operative infection risk. One should distinguish those from the bio-compatible bone substitutes used to fill bony defects.

3.3.8
Artefacts

Bone defects and abnormalities have to be distinguished from artefacts. The latter are structures or appearances that are only present on the radiograph and are produced by an artificial means. If the identity of the artefact cannot be established, additional radiographs of the region should be obtained. Digital radiography allows an easy differential diagnosis.

3.4
A Practical Guide for Pre-Operative Planning

This paragraph sets out to be a practical guide for the clinician who is confronted with a patient who needs rehabilitation by means of endosseous implants. It provides practical details for different imaging procedures in different situations.

3.4.1
Implant Placement in the Edentulous Mandible

When planning implant placement in an edentulous mandible, one needs information on the bone height in the anterior region. Implants are normally placed in between the mental foramina, where bone quality and quantity are usually sufficient and where no critical anatomic structures interfere. A panoramic radiograph is therefore the method of choice. One should however take into account the horizontal and vertical magnification error. It is suggested to measure the radiographic bone height and divide it by the average magnification factor of 1.25. Another possibility is the use of metal markers of known dimensions and calculate the magnification in that particular area (see § 2.2). When bone height is less than 10 mm, CT scan evaluation is recommended to obtain a more detailed and accurate information on the remaining bone.

3.4.2
Implant Placement in the Maxilla or Posterior Mandible

The CT scan is still the technique of choice for optimal planning of implant placement either in the maxilla or the posterior mandible. By inspecting the scout view, an overview of the CT sections is provided (Fig. 3.8). Conventional (incremental) CT scanning uses slices of 2 mm of thickness, while 1-mm slices are usually available with spiral CT scanning.

In both instances, axial and cross-sectional views can be interpreted. Axial views are interpreted first to evaluate the degree of bone mineralisation, to obtain an estimate of the available bone height and the location and extension of the anatomic structures. Bone pathology is also best observed on these direct images. Afterwards,

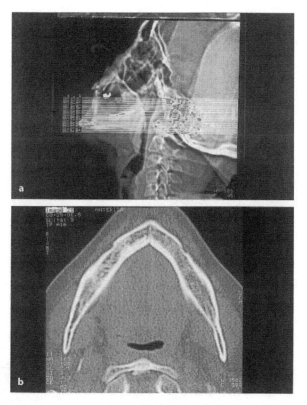

Fig. 3.8. The scout view presented with the CT scan images provides an overview of the CT sections **(a)**. One of the axial scan sections is demonstrated **(b)** (from the Department of Radiology, University Hospital Gasthuisberg, Leuven, Belgium)

cross-sectional views produced by computer software at the proposed implant sites can be inspected. To assess whether implant placement would be possible, it is recommended to use a transparent template with the relative lengths and diameters of the commercially available implant system (Fig. 3.9). By superposition of the template on the cross-sectional CT images of the jaw bone and taking into account the eventual magnification factor – normally CT images are life-size – the optimal lengths and axes are determined for implant placement. One should keep in mind the diameter of the implant. Depending on the diameter of the implant used, the same implant should fit within two or more cross-sectional views to avoid fenestrations, dehiscenses or damage to anatomic structures (Fig. 3.10). When defining the optimal implant length, one must use the accuracy of the radiographic technique applied. For conventional tomography and computer tomography, discrepancies between measured and actual bone height are on average 0.4–0.5 mm (Petrowski et al. 1989; Quirynen et al. 1990). Since measurement errors are in the range of 1 mm, it is recommended to keep a safety margin of about 1–2 mm from the mandibular canal (Klinge et al. 1989) or other less critical anatomic structures (sinus and nasal floor, incisive canal).

Not only the implant dimensions and orientation are important. Successful integration is also dependent on the bone quality and the primary stability (van Steenberghe et al. 1995). Efforts should be made to obtain a (bi)cortical contact with the

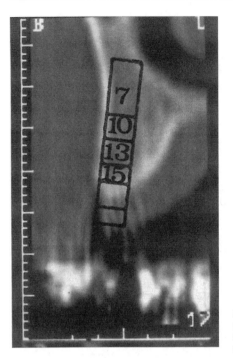

Fig. 3.9. A transparent template is superposed on a cross-sectional image of the edentulous maxilla to determine the optimal implant length and axis. Here a 15-mm implant could be installed

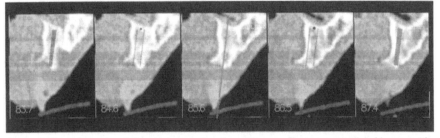

Fig. 3.10. The 3-dimensional planning system based on CT scans, allows cross-sectional images with a 0.4 mm interval. When interactively placing a 3.75 mm diameter implant in the 3-D images on the computer screen, its placement can be controlled on several cross-sectional images (from the Laboratory of Medical Imaging Research, Department of Electrical Engineering, ESAT, Department of Radiology, University Hospital Gasthuisberg, Leuven, Belgium)

implant. Placement of the implant in poor quality trabecular bone (very low density) should be avoided when possible. The density of the local bone can be defined by means of the Hounsfield density scale. On the Hounsfield scale air has a relative density of -1000, water is 0 and extreme dense bone $+1000$. The interpretation of this density measure is dependent on the applied imaging parameters and the choice of the density window. One should attempt to visualise bone as well as nervous tissue. Nerve bundles have an important amount of fatty tissue and a score from 0 to -100 and should be included in the density window as such that they become visual. An important factor to consider is the jaw bone quality around the planned implant location. Such measurements are especially important in the upper jaw with a poor bone quality (Duckmanton et al. 1994). On a special request, the mean density of a particular region of the jaw can be assessed by making Hounsfield densitometric readings. Usually, density readings of an area of 1.0 mm^2 are made at the planned implant site, at a position midway between the bone crest and for example the floor of the sinus. The densitometric readings will vary in relationship to the contrast and brightness settings on the CT equipment and must be interpreted as relative values rather than absolute values. For a particular CT equipment or a particular clinical team, a reference population should be built up, providing a range of densitometric readings with a high predictability for a successful clinical outcome.

3.4.3
Single Tooth Replacement

Regularly single implant placement is planned while the tooth to be replaced is still in place. This also applies to the replacement of several teeth especially in the anterior region. It is difficult to predict what the bone resorption will be after tooth extraction. It depends on a variety of factors such as the degree of loss of attachment and the surgical technique (hermetic closure or not). Tomographs or reformatted CT scan images revealing the vestibulo-oral plane allow the clinician to evaluate the bone apical to the teeth to be extracted and cautiously conclude whether enough bone will remain or not. One must realise that the long axis of the tooth can often not be followed during the insertion of the implant for a variety of reasons:

- to avoid an unaesthetic implant position
- to achieve a good primary stability at insertion (no fenestrations)
- to obtain contact with the cortex
- to aim for occlusion with the antagonistic teeth
- to allow a proper lip support

Intra-oral radiographs after tooth extraction are essential before planning to install implants in previous extraction wounds. It is not easy to decide when this radiograph should be taken. When the tooth to be extracted has a quite normal periodontal bone level, implant installation must be delayed 3 to 4 months after careful extraction, curettage and primary closure of the extraction wound. When only 1/3 of the root length remains surrounded by bone, implants may be installed as soon as 1 month after extraction. Immediate implant installation is another alternative, involving more complications, but still offering a high success rate.

3.4.4
Pre-Prosthetic Planning

Implant placement should best be performed taking into account both surgical and prosthetic aspects. The anatomic structures, the biomechanical requirements and aesthetic demands should all be considered. Pre-operative information from the radiographic evaluation and prosthetic requirements can be transferred to a surgical template. One way to combine both anatomic and prosthetic aspects is to provide radiopaque markers on the prosthesis and to take a radiograph with the prosthesis in situ. In this manner, it may be possible to establish the relationship between bone, prosthesis and tooth location. For conventional tomography, metal markers are usually placed in a reference splint at potential implant sites (Stella and Tharanon 1990; Lee and Morgano 1994; Ismail et al. 1995).

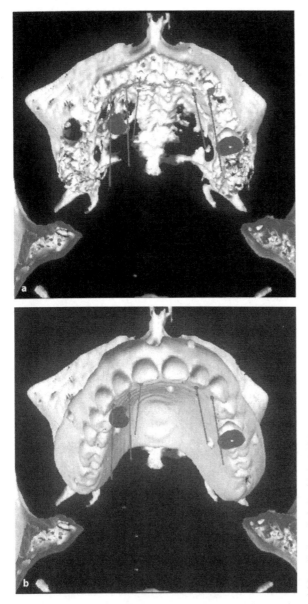

Fig. 3.11. A 3-dimensional visualisation of the jaw bone without (a) and with (b) the removable prosthesis, which was visualised by applying gutta percha markers on the prosthesis. The prosthesis remained in place during the scanning procedure. Afterwards, it was separately scanned with low energy to become radiographically visible and integrated in the 3-D image of the jaw by fusion on the basis of the gutta percha markers (from the Laboratory of Medical Imaging Research, Department of Electrical Engineering, ESAT, Department of Radiology, University Hospital Gasthuisberg, Leuven, Belgium)

Stent marker materials for CT scanning range from simple types such as small (2 mm) metal spheres or gutta percha to more sophisticated materials, such as prosthetic teeth painted with a radiopaque coating or prostheses impregnated with radiopaque materials.

Borrow and Smith (1996) evaluated 7 different markers for pre-operative planning of implant placement by means of CT scan:

- 5-mm lead or steel spheres
- 2-mm steel spheres
- gutta percha markers on an acrylic stent
- barium sulphate mixed with varnish to coat the denture
- radiopaque prosthetic teeth (7 g BaSO$_4$ in 5 ml varnish)
- radiopaque prosthetic teeth (made from a mixture of BaSO$_4$ 5% with acrylic material)
- radiopaque prosthetic teeth with gutta percha filled holes to indicate the gingival border
- radiopaque prosthetic teeth with non-filled holes within the teeth at potential implant sites

Steel spheres, especially the larger ones, generate substantial artefacts. Gutta percha (contains BaSO$_4$) is an excellent moderately radiopaque marker, which is not obscured by artefacts (Fig. 3.11). Painting teeth with a radiopaque coating is preferred to the fabrication of radiopaque teeth, since one can easily use the existing prosthesis (Fig. 3.12). Information on the orientation and location of the teeth on the radiographs allows to optimise the pre-operative planning for implant placement. Thus, it is possible to consider bone quantity, the anatomic structures, the aesthetic and biomechanical aspects and use all these data to manufacture the surgical template with concavities at the implant sites to guide the drilling instruments. A practical approach is to consider a stent with radiopaque material for the CT scan and modify

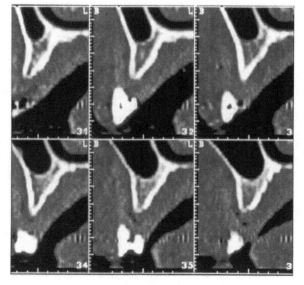

Fig. 3.12. Barium sulphate mixed with varnish is used to coat the denture teeth, prior to scanning. It enables a clear visualisation of the acrylic teeth on the cross-sectional images of the CT scan (from the Department of Radiology, University Hospital Gasthuisberg, Leuven, Belgium)

this stent afterwards to guide the surgical placement of implants (Lima Verde and Morgano 1993). In any case, one should try to transfer CT scan data to surgical data using anatomic landmarks as reference points (Karellos and Zouras 1993). Some authors recommend the use of drilling ducts within the surgical template (Modica et al. 1991), but this leads to the risk that the duct determines too strictly the implant placement and that cooling and visibility become insufficient.

3.4.5
Conclusions

The rehabilitation of the (partially) edentulous jaw bone by means of endosseous implants is determined by the result of careful pre-operative examination using the appropriate radiographic technique. Quite often, a compromise between optimal surgical and optimal prosthetic implant placement is needed. Pre-operative consultation should be organised between surgeon and restorative dentist. This can be done by phone or eventually by network. Data of the proposed implant sites should be transferred to a surgical template, to help determining implant axes during surgery.

Table 3.1. Guidelines for choosing the appropriate imaging technique during pre-operative planning of implant placement

Indication		Technique[1]	Execution
# implants per edentulous region	location	technique of choice[2] (alternative technique)	
1 implant	single tooth replacement (frontal region, after extraction)	1 intra-oral radiograph paralleling technique	dentist
	but: extreme bone resorption; buccal concavity; enlarged foramen incisivum; proximity sinus maxillaris	incremental CT (conventional tomograph)	radiologist
2 implants	edentulous anterior mandible (between mental foramina)	panoramic radiograph	dentist/ radiologist
	partially edentulous anterior mandible	2 intra-oral radiographs	dentist
	posterior mandible	incremental CT (spiral CT)	radiologist
	maxilla	incremental CT (spiral CT)	radiologist
> 2 implants	anterior mandible (between mental foramina)	panoramic radiograph	dentist/ radiologist
	posterior mandible	3-D CT – spiral CT (incremental CT)	radiologist
	maxilla	3-D CT – spiral CT (incremental CT)	radiologist
implants + complex surgery in maxillo-facial area	mandible/maxilla	stereolithography – 3-D CT	radiologist

[1] The appropriate technique is determined by its diagnostic output, outweighing the radiation dose against the information obtained

[2] Whenever the technique of choice is not available, one can choose the alternative technique presented in between brackets

Part II

Radiographic Follow-Up of Endosseous Implants

Radiographic Follow-Up of Endosseous Implants

Bone apposition has been shown at the histological level on a variety of endosseous implant surfaces. According to Søballe (1993), implant fixation is dependent on a number of variables: modification in the prosthetic and/or implant design, changes in the host bone status, adjuvant therapies or adaptations for mechanical stabilisation (Table II.1).

Bone apposition should not be, although it often is, called osseointegration. The latter term introduced by Brånemark also implies the stability of the bone over time. An implant is said to be osseointegrated if there is no progressive relative motion of living bone and implant under functional levels and types of loading for the entire life of the patient (Rydevik et al. 1991). It implies a close bone apposition to the implant

Table II.1. Implant fixation in orthopaedics is dependent on a number of variables (modified from Søballe 1993)

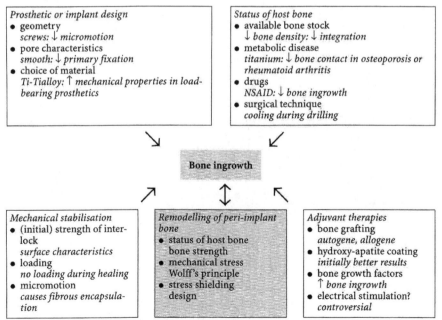

surface with continuous remodelling of the supporting bone. It means the mainte-
nance over the years of:

- a stable marginal bone height
- an intimate bone to implant contact around the entire contour

The long-term clinical success of endosseous implants which achieve osseointegration has been reported extensively (Albrektsson et al. 1988; Adell et al. 1990).

Although one cannot confirm at the radiographic level whether this bone apposition exists at the histological level, the presence of a peri-implant radiolucency certainly proves a lack of bone apposition. Lack of intimate bone apposition can also be
identified by clinical symptoms (mobility, unmanageable pain, infection, …)
(Albrektsson et al. 1986).

Success in implant treatment is a primary concern of patient, clinician and third par-
ties such as insurance companies and governments. This illustrates the need for a precise
definition of implant success. Different criteria and standards have been proposed and
are often associated with a radiographic follow-up to evaluate the peri-implant bone
level and to detect a peri-implant radiolucency in case of implant failure (Albrektsson et
al. 1986; Smith and Zarb 1989). The 1978 National Institutes of Health Harvard Consensus
Development Conference provided the first widely sourced criteria for implant success.
An objective criterion was formulated as follows: "bone loss no greater that $1/3$ of the vertical height of the implant, with absence of symptoms and functionally stable after 5
years" (Schnitman and Schulman 1980). One should realise that the published work from
Brånemark et al. (1977; 10 years data) was omitted from this meeting. Thus a stable marginal bone level was still considered unachievable. This kind of criterion may be appropriate for teeth but not for implants, where dealing with a variety of implant lengths
(Chaytor 1993). More stringent criteria were proposed in 1986 and 1992. Albrektsson et al.
(1986) stated that "vertical bone loss should be less than 0.2 mm annually following the
implant's first year of service". The success criteria were listed as follows:

- absence of a continuous radiolucency
- no clinical mobility
- remodelling of 0.9 – 1.6 mm during the first year
- remodelling rate of 0.1 mm during the following years

The proposal by Albrektsson and Zarb (1993) left the mean annual changes at 0.2 mm,
but considered implant location as an important factor and therefore made a distinction between anterior and posterior zones.

Naert et al. (1992) defined failure of an implant as follows:

- "slightest" sign of mobility
- peri-implant radiolucency
- pain or infection

Nevertheless, definition of success by means of clinical criteria has certain limitations. Albrektsson and Jacobsson (1987) stated that the difference between cell size
and optimal resolution capacity of radiography is more than 10-fold and clinical
radiographs cannot be used as an evidence of osseointegration. The best documentation of success may then be the follow-up of the individual patient during decades
and against strict criteria for success (van Steenberghe 1997).

Radiography is one of the most frequently used diagnostic procedures in patients with endosseous implants. It enables to visualise implant failure, improper placement of an implant and/or violation of important anatomic structures. Currently the following radiographic parameters may be used for assessment of peri-implant bone:

Bone quantity
- bone quantity grading (McKinney et al. 1983; Nasr and Meffert 1993)
- analogue measurements of bone level (Hollender and Rockler 1980)
- computer-assisted bone level assessment (Weber et al. 1992)

Bone quality
- bone quality grading (Adell et al. 1986)

Since the number of radiographic examinations has to be limited, there is a need for other clinical parameters in the evaluation of implant assessment.

The validity and reliability of each of these techniques will be reviewed in the chapters below. Chapter 4 will concentrate on bone quantity around implants, chapter 5 on bone quality. Finally, chapter 6 will provide us with radiographic appearances of complications and/or failures.

Bone Quantity

4.1
Methodologies for Assessment of Alveolar Bone Quantity

Over the past two decades, much research has been carried out to develop radiographic methods that improve the ability to detect and measure the jaw bone level. A conventional intra-oral radiograph is a relatively crude tool to quantify and qualify the jaw bone due to:

- variations in projection geometry
- variations in contrast and density of the radiographs
- two-dimensional nature of the radiographic image (overlapping of anatomic structures)
- uncontrolled film processing
- variability in peak kilovoltage (kVp) / exposure time

Information on the bone level can be obtained through planimetric (Nielsen et al. 1980) and linear measurements. The latter are far more popular and different ways of expressing such linear measurements have been suggested:

- relative, proportional to tooth or root length (Schei et al. 1959) (Fig. 4.1)
- absolute, in mm regardless of image magnification (Hollender et al. 1980)
- absolute, in mm with correction of the calculated (Weiss and Ronen 1977) or corrected magnification (Eggen 1976; Larheim and Eggen 1982)

Early attempts to compensate for angular discrepancies include the use of a radiographic grid. When the radiograph is exposed, the 1-mm grid is superimposed on the radiographic image of the anatomic area of interest providing a reference for measurement of bone height. Although the technique is simple to use, results are misleading. Since the grid is placed directly on the film, the image of the grid does not distort, while the image of the bone is elongated or foreshortened.

The Schei ruler is a one-dimensional method for the compensation of geometric discrepancies (Schei et al. 1959). Bone height is expressed as a ratio of the root length to compensate for distortion of the image. The classical Schei ruler has only 5 or 10 gradations with which the clinician can grade the extent of the bone loss. The latter implies that 20 or 10 % of the bone must have been lost before detection occurs. This problem has been circumvented by introducing digitising devices which may detect bone changes of 1.5 % (Jeffcoat and Williams 1984). Another disadvantage of the original Schei ruler is that it provides only a relative measure of the bone height. By means of algorithms, angulation errors are partly corrected and absolute measurements can be provided (Jeffcoat et al. 1984).

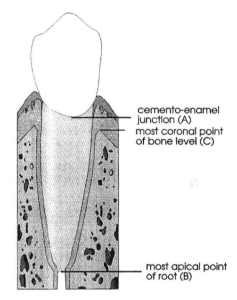

cemento-enamel
junction (A)
most coronal point
of bone level (C)

most apical point
of root (B)

Fig. 4.1. The relative bone level is calculated as the vertical distance between the marginal bone level (C) and the root apex (B) proportionally to the distance between the cemento-enamel junction (A) and the root apex (B)

Another alternative is to utilise the radiographic view that produces minimal distortion of the tooth-bone height relationship. Compared to the conventional bisecting-angle technique, a paralleling technique, preferably with a long cone, offers more diagnostic information. The use of a long cone is based on the following reasoning. When placing the film in parallel to the teeth, the object-film distance increases, resulting in a decreased sharpness of the image (Fig. 4.2). It can be enhanced again by increasing the focus-object distance (Van Aken 1969). Because the intensity of the x-ray beam decreases with distance, the intensity and the voltage have to be enhanced (e. g. 15 mA – 90 kVp). The technique reduces the patient irradiation sensibly due to

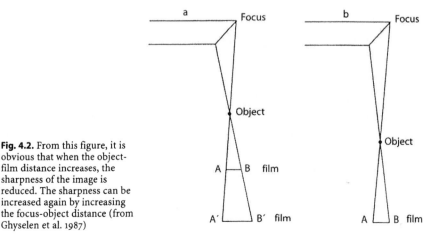

Fig. 4.2. From this figure, it is obvious that when the object-film distance increases, the sharpness of the image is reduced. The sharpness can be increased again by increasing the focus-object distance (from Ghyselen et al. 1987)

collimation, filtration, the higher kilovoltage and the use of a long cone. Theoretically, the intra-oral radiograph could supply information on the horizontal and vertical dimensions of the jaw bone, but practically the two-dimensional nature of a single radiograph involves distortion and overlapping of anatomical structures.

4.2
Methodologies for Assessment of Peri-Implant Bone Quantity

4.2.1
Conventional Intra-Oral Radiography

The nature of the bone-implant interface can only be revealed at a histological level. Clinically, non-invasive techniques are needed to assess implant success or failure (= fibrous tissue interposed between implant and bone). The radiographic evaluation usually takes place for the first time at abutment installation (two-stage implant system), due to the potential effect of radiation on bone healing around the implant. Based on long-term clinical studies and supported by animal studies, clinical healing times for osseointegration are a minimum of 3 months for dense bone and 6 months for cancellous bone (Adell 1992). During this period radiographs are not informative and since bone healing could be depressed by the radiation effects clinicians should refrain from it. For one-stage implants there can be a need for earlier radiographic diagnosis.

Implants offer a number of advantages in radiological interpretation compared to teeth (Fig. 4.3).

An implant offers the possibility to use reliable reference points, such as the top of the abutment or the implant-abutment junction in the case of a two-stage implant system. Secondly, the radiopacity of many metallic implants implies a better contrast with the surrounding structures. Indeed, radiographic images of titanium implants will exhibit a uniform radiopacity with minimal peripheral burn-out. Burn-out phenomena denoted as the "Mach bands" are visual phenomena with borders of adjacent areas giving larger density differences than really exist (Ratliff 1965). In areas of diminished dimensions, the burn-out will be more pronounced. In Brånemark implants (Brånemark System, Nobel Biocare, Gothenburg, Sweden) for example, the latter phenomenon gives the impression of a conical shape in the apical region, where the volume of the peripheral part is less than that of the main part due to the four ver-

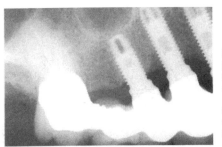

Fig. 4.3. The advantages of implants for radiographic interpretation are:
● reliable reference points
● better contrast with the surrounding structures
● known density (reference to bone density)
● known dimensions (correction factor)
● superimposition of implants (subsequent radiographs

tical cuts (Sewerin 1992). When these cuts are situated laterally on the radiograph, the impression of a conical aspect will be intensified. Burn-out phenomena have to be differentiated from the diagnosis of fibrous encapsulation (Sewerin 1992).

Thirdly, the known density of the metallic implants can be used for radiographic evaluation of the density of surrounding bone.

Fourthly, the known implant dimensions can be used for calculating the correction factor for angulations.

Finally, superimposition of metallic implants on lateral cephalograms can be used to monitor craniofacial changes. This corresponds well to the method used by Björk in orthodontics where small metallic implants are visualised through lateral cephalograms to measure the mandibular remodelling (Baumrind et al. 1992). Overall superimposition of metallic implants and superimposition of mandibular anatomic structures according to the common "best fit" rule, yields differences in linear measurements smaller than 1 mm. Nevertheless, for case measurements, results from superimposition methods vary considerably, noting that the aforementioned method can be used for assessing a general remodelling pattern but not for the individual patient (Baumrind et al. 1992).

Panoramic radiographs cannot be used to describe in detail the extent of peri-implant defects (Fig. 4.4). They can only be used for a more subjective description of bony defects around endosseous implants (Mericske-Stern et al. 1994). Further developments in panoramic radiography, especially with respect to digital imaging may increase their potential use in longitudinal clinical evaluation of oral implants.

Grading systems have been introduced to assess peri-implant bone levels and implant success over time (Schnitman et al. 1980). The radiographic indices are how-

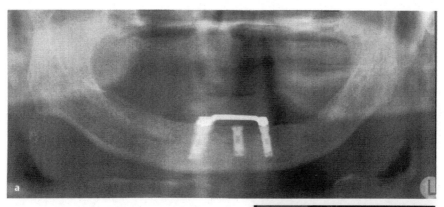

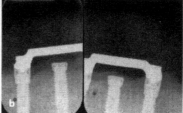

Fig. 4.4. Panoramic radiographs of an edentulous patient, who has been rehabilitated by means of screw-shaped titanium implants connected by a bar and supporting an overdenture in the lower jaw **(a)**. A much more detailed image of the peri-implant bone is seen on the intra-oral radiographs using the long-cone paralleling technique **(b)**. The "sleeping" implant in the middle was installed because of the experimental set-up

ever non-linear and discontinuous, which implies that they remain within a certain grade, even though important osseous changes can occur. Although the methodological studies indicate their clinical validity, such indices seem seldom applied. McKinney et al. (1983) proposed the following index:

0 = no radiographic evidence of bone resorption around the implant
1 = slight resorption (< 0.5 mm)
2 = moderate resorption (0.5 – 2 mm)
3 = severe resorption (> 2 mm)
4 = radicular radiolucency, having a width of 1.5 mm and along more than 1/3 of the root surface

Nasr and Meffert (1993) proposed an easy comprehensive reference guide for evaluating implant success on standardised long-cone radiographs. They denoted interproximal marginal bone loss in percentages relative to the implant body length using index scores ranging from 0 to 6:

0 = marginal bone loss extending to 0 – 5 % of implant length
1 =   > 5 up to 10 %
2 =   > 10 up to 15 %
3 =   > 15 up to 20 %
4 =   > 20 up to 25 %
5 =   > 25 up to 30 %
6 =   > 30 %

One should realise that involving the implant length as a success criterion has important consequences. Although the same marginal bone loss occurs, a shorter implant will sooner be considered as failed than a longer one (Fig. 4.5).

Some more detailed grading could be obtained by adding a positive or negative sign to the grade for values above or below the mean of the interval score. For bone loss with grade 1 (> 5 – 10 %), the latter implies that a positive sign is added (1+) when bone loss exceeds 7.5 %. A negative sign is added (1–) for values < 7.5 %. This index was claimed to be more comprehensive to compare different implant lengths and/or systems. But this advantage might also be a major problem, because the variety of implant lengths, diameters and designs may involve very different bone remodelling patterns. Another problem with this index is that it can only be used for smaller implants and often not for maxillary implants, because of the difficulty of parallel projection geometry between implant, film and x-ray beam. It is evident that absolute changes in marginal bone level should be monitored.

For accurate peri-implant bone level assessment, a strict paralleling technique is essential, especially for imaging screw-shaped implants. Even at small deviations (5 °), significant defects may be occluded (Hollender and Rockler 1980). The parallel long-cone intra-oral radiographs are offering a precise image of the jaw bone structures and of the bone height (Fig. 4.6). Early standardised procedures to evaluate peri-implant bone were described by Hollender and Rockler (1980) and Strid (1985 a+b). Since then, different studies have been carried out using a variety of radio-

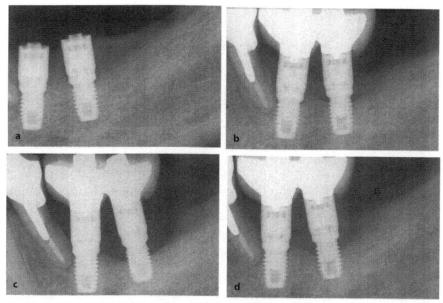

Fig. 4.5. Intra-oral radiographs of two short implants with substantial bone loss over an 4-year time, period (**a**: year 1; **b**: year 3; **c**: year 5) because of an unfavourable superstructure / implant length relationship. At year 7 (**d**) bone loss could be arrested.

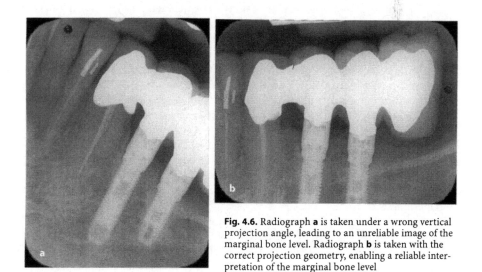

Fig. 4.6. Radiograph **a** is taken under a wrong vertical projection angle, leading to an unreliable image of the marginal bone level. Radiograph **b** is taken with the correct projection geometry, enabling a reliable interpretation of the marginal bone level

graphic parameters (for review see Brägger 1994). A film holder (Eggen 1969) can be used for standardised serial identical stereopairs of radiographs with parallel projection (Fig. 4.7). If the implant is screw-shaped, marginal bone changes can be registered mesially and distally of the implants, resulting in measuring units half of the

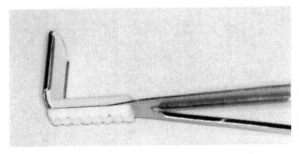

Fig. 4.7. An Eggen holder can be used for paralleling radiography, which facilitates the positioning of the x-ray tube under different horizontal projection angles

interthread distance. The accuracy of this method with e.g. Brånemark implants (0.6 mm interthread distance) is 0.3 mm.

The absence of the periodontal ligament space around implants, improves the identification of the peri-implant bone level (Larheim and Eggen 1982). It is also found that the use of an individual impression to allow a precise replacement of the Eggen holder improved the accuracy of the method. This technique has a measurement error ($\sqrt{\Sigma d^2 / 2n}$) of 0.21 mm for peri-implant bone height and 0.24 mm for periodontal bone height (d = difference between duplicate measurements; n = total number of duplicate measurements). The improved measurements for peri-implant bone height can be related to the aforementioned radiographic advantages of implant configuration.

For clinical practice however, identical exposure geometry, needed for follow-up of peri-implant bone level, remains very difficult to obtain. By means of the long-cone paralleling technique and a paralleling device (e.g. Rinn film holder, Rinn Corporation, Elgin, IL, USA) (Fig. 4.8), the distance between a reference point and the marginal bone level around implants can be assessed with great accuracy using a sliding calliper (Quirynen et al. 1991b). When using this technique for bone height measurements around both threaded and cylindrical implants on intra-oral radiographs, a mean inter-examiner difference of 0.09 – 0.16 mm can be established (Quirynen et al. 1992a).

With the technique described by el Charkawi (1989) standardised serial intra-oral radiographs are obtained to measure changes of bone level around titanium plasma-sprayed screw-shaped implants placed in the mandibular symphyseal region. A template of autopolymerising acrylic resin is made to hold the film parallel to the implants and is connected to a standard long tube through a paralleling device. This procedure assures constant focus-film and implant-film distances throughout all exposures. The distance from the bottom of the superstructure to the top of the residual ridge is measured with a sliding calliper. This technique has major drawbacks. The fact that 4 implants (used to support an overdenture) are placed on one radiograph questions the parallelity of the radiograph. It is hard to have a perfect parallel installation of 4 implants in the mandible. To have them projected on one radiograph certainly involves deformation due to the curvature of the mandible.

Cox and Pharoah (1986) described a film holder device attached to the abutments, after removal of the superstructure. Vertical angulation errors can be eliminated by using a long transfer coping screw, that fits tightly into a hole in the intra-oral hori-

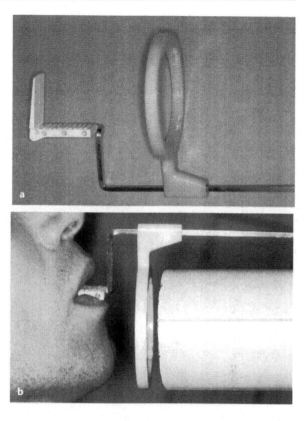

Fig. 4.8. The Rinn film holder facilitates an optimal projection geometry for paralleling radiography. **a** Film holder for the frontal region. **b** Film holder in place for paralleling radiography of the lower incisors

zontal portion of the holder (Cox and Pharoah 1986). These arrangements permit an almost parallel projection geometry and can be used for post-operative radiological evaluation of small bone changes (Meijer et al. 1992; Pharoah 1993), without being necessary to depict the whole implant length (Cox and Pharoah 1986). Nevertheless, because these holders require the detachment of the fixed prosthesis, their application should be limited to overdentures, urgent diagnostic needs or longitudinal research. Furthermore, the 2-dimensional image of the 3-dimensional structures remains a major drawback and may lead to masking of intra-bony defects or misinterpretation of buccolingual bone level differences. One could suggest to use stereoscopic radiography to provide a better estimate of the bone level and/or defect around implants. However, such images remain only qualitative (Tammisalo et al. 1992; Frederiksen 1995).

In general, assessment of changes in peri-implant bone level has the following limitations:

- only interproximal aspects can be evaluated
- mesial and distal bone level changes are usually averaged for statistics
- reporting the mean annual change in peri-implant bone height is more valuable for documentation of success of an implant system than for clinical patient monitoring

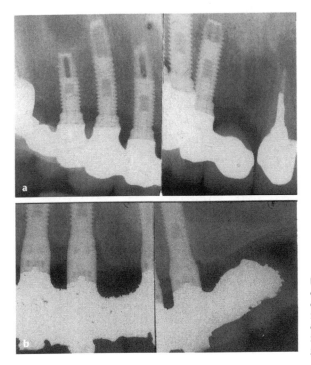

Fig. 4.9. Maxillary implants extending into the palate are often distorted (**a**). It is better to focus on the region of interest, e. g. the coronal part of the implant to evaluate the marginal bone level (**b**)

For the interpretation of bone fill of peri-implant bone defects by implantable materials a lack of standardised serial measurements is often noticed (Becker et al. 1994). These bony defects certainly require an accurate quantity and even more precise quality grading, which can only be accomplished by using subtraction radiography (Galgut et al. 1991).

Since it is often cumbersome to use bite holders to reproduce previous projection angles, it may be advantageous that the implant geometry offers the possibility to evaluate the projection geometry on the radiographic image. By a strictly parallel geometry between film, radiation beam and implant axis, the threaded surface of a screw-type implant is represented on a 2-dimensional image (Sewerin 1991a). This condition may sometimes be difficult to obtain because of the inclination of the implant and the anatomy of the patient. Maxillary implants extending in the vertical direction above the hard palate cannot be imaged entirely without distortions. In these cases it is better to focus on the region of interest (the bone margin) instead of imaging the whole implant (Fig. 4.9). In fact, there is only a need to visualise the coronal part of the implant if one chooses to express the marginal bone loss as an absolute value rather than a proportion of the total implant length. This is more easy to obtain and more meaningful. Recently, it has been suggested to apply narrow-beam radiography when paralleling radiography is almost impossible (Svenson and Palmqvist 1996). It provides images from 4 slightly different projection angles, to obtain a stereoscopic effect. Unfortunately, this technique is only available in a very limited number of centres.

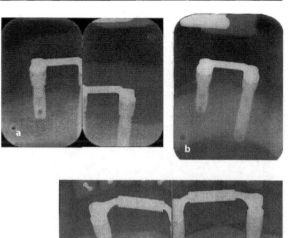

Fig. 4.10. When the threads of screw-shaped implants are clearly visible **(a)**, the correct projection geometry has been applied. Otherwise threads are obscured **(b)**

Fig. 4.11. For cylindrical implants, it is difficult to find any reference to control the projection geometry

When taking radiographs of an extremely resorbed mandible, it is often impossible to place the film intra-orally because of the interference of the floor of the mouth. An extra-oral film placement by means of a rigid plastic holder parallel and attached to the rectangular collimator may be used (Hollender and Rockler 1980). Even with a correct projection geometry, the radiographic identification of the bone level surrounding the implant may be insufficient. It remains possible that parts of the superimposed bone are at a higher level than the implant neck. In the follow-up, horizontal angulation of the x-ray beam may thus lead to a false interpretation of the peri-implant bone level. It has to be stressed that the contact area between implant and bone depicted on a radiograph only represents a small amount of the total peri-implant bone level (Sewerin 1992).

Because different implants mostly have different angulations, imaging must be individualised. An intra-oral view or a panoramic radiograph may supply information on the implant angulations. The threads of screw-shaped implants can be used in the interpretation of angular deviations (Fig. 4.10). For cylindrical implants, radiographic evaluation of the angular deviation is less obvious (Fig. 4.11). Deviations smaller than 7° are tolerable (Hollender 1992). But a deviation of 1° results in a misinterpretation of the marginal bone height of at least 0.1 mm (Sewerin 1990). It has even been stated that in spite of all achievements regarding the validity and reliability of bone height measurements, an accuracy below 0.2 mm cannot be obtained even with optimum imaging techniques (Benn 1992).

About 13° of angular deviation from the ideal totally obscures the threads. Between 7 and 13°, correction can be made on the basis of the blurring of the threads by changing the film inclination in a vertical direction. Due to the right-handed threads of screw-shaped implants, the threadings at the right side will be obscured when the implant is imaged from a coronal direction. When the implant is seen from an apical direction, threadings on the left side will be occluded. While vertical angulations can be easily determined, horizontal rotation is hard to assess. A 0° rotation

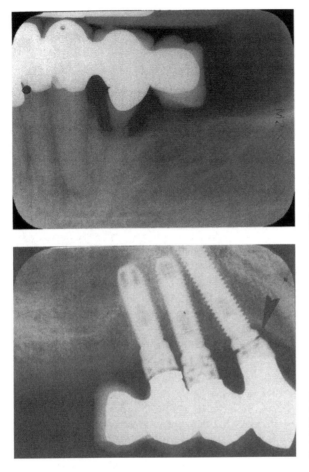

Fig. 4.12. Intra-oral radiograph of aluminium oxide implant, indicating that it is not that easy to discriminate it from bone

Fig. 4.13. For two stage-implants, an intra-oral radiograph is taken under an optimal projection geometry, also to detect eventual slits between implant and abutment (arrow)

and angulation is characterised by a complete image of the implant characteristics (e.g. perforation in apical third). At a different rotation, left or right rotation can hardly be distinguished.

Cylindrical titanium implants (e.g. implant, IMZ, Friatec AG, Mannheim, Germany) show a symmetric image with a good radiopacity. Evaluation of the vertical angulation allows only a crude estimation. The rounded base of the IMZ implant for example looks similar at all vertical angulations and is of no help. The four vertical slits in the apical third offer a good opportunity for estimation of the rotation and the angulation, but the inconstant radiographic image may be a disturbing factor (Sewerin 1991b).

Implant design influences image density and image pattern (Sewerin 1991b). Many implants exhibit perforations, grooves, cuts, vents, cores and threads, which permit specific implant identification but also act as disturbing factors in image interpretation (Sewerin 1991b). Solid metallic implants are easily identified, whereas ceramic implants (aluminium oxide, hydroxy-apatite) are less discernible (Sewerin 1991b)(Fig. 4.12). Radiolucent zones around an implant clearly indicate fibrous tissue anchorage, but the lack of such zones is not sufficient proof of bone apposition (Albrektsson and Jacobsson 1987). Furthermore, the detection of non-osseointegration should be distinguished from the typical Mach bands (see § 4.2.1) (Hollender 1992).

An optimal projection geometry is also necessary to evaluate slits of the implant-abutment connection. Slits of 0.1 mm may be obscured by deviations of 5° only (Sewerin 1989) (Fig. 4.13).

4.2.2
Computerised Analysis of Bone Quantity

Conventional intra-oral radiographs seem to offer a high diagnostic specificity but a rather low sensitivity in detecting periodontal lesions. One of the major difficulties is the discrimination of a lesion against a background of superimposed anatomic structures. Digitalisation and subtraction techniques are able to increase the sensitivity of the radiographs to even minute changes of the bone. During digital conversion of a radiograph, the information contained in an image is decomposed into bits (binary digits), positioned into a matrix (for review see Wenzel 1993). Each point in this matrix is termed a pixel (picture element), which is the smallest information unit in the image. Each pixel corresponds to a shade of grey. Nowadays, 256 grey shades are usually available ranging from 0 (=black) to 255 (=white). The smaller the pixel, the higher the resolution and the more details that can be displayed. In a digital image, contrast can be enhanced by scaling and transforming the input pixels in order to utilise all possible grey shades defined by the digital system. Underexposed conventional radiographs can thus be digitally enhanced, obtaining an improved contrast and density. Edge enhancement sharpens the edges of imaged structures by filtering procedures to facilitate the detection of boundaries between healthy and diseased areas. It improves image quality and increases the diagnostic information. Subtraction involves superimposition of two subsequent radiographs and elimination of the identical structures (anatomic noise). Colour enhancement is helping to identify and highlight bone with the same densities by replacing specific grey level values with colour. Digital subtraction has been shown to be superior to conventional radiography in detecting small marginal alveolar bone changes (for review see Wenzel 1993). Digital analysis and subtraction seems also suitable for evaluating peri-implant bone level changes, since implants offer certain advantages over teeth:

- fixed reference points on the implant
- known dimensions
- known density
- high contrast with surrounding bone

Standardised projection geometry is a prerequisite for longitudinal observation of the peri-implant bone level, especially with regard to digitalisation and subtraction. By means of specially designed film holders, which can be attached to the abutments, reproducible radiographs may be obtained and subtraction radiography may be performed to detect bone level changes over time (Meijer et al. 1992). Standardised radiographs may also be obtained by using film holders and individual bite blocks (Weber et al. 1992).

Several recipes for bone height determination were proposed which are specific for oral endosseous implants. Meijer et al. (1993) introduced a technique which includes scanning of the radiographs with a CCD camera for analogue to digital conversion (256 grey levels). Afterwards, contrast is enhanced and points are interactively determined on the edge of the implant for determining the bone level. Reproducibility of duplicate measurements reveals a measurement error of 0.55 mm ($\sqrt{\Sigma d^2/ 2n}$). The error is somewhat better than for a magnifying glass with measuring scale (0.80 mm) or the usage of a digital sliding calliper (0.75 mm).

Reddy et al. (1992) developed a reproducible method for measurement of bone support around oral implants, using a grid projected on the implant. The grid is defined by the known dimensions of the implant, compensating for both vertical and horizontal projection distortions. Thus, standardised radiographs are not required. The software automatically detects the implant edge. Interactively, the bone edge has to be indicated at each point were the grid intersects the implant. Thus, the actual size of the defect is automatically calculated. Reproducibility of the method is expressed by the standard deviation of repeated measurements ($n = 5$), being 0.08 mm for root form implants and 0.19 mm for blade form implants.

Weber et al. (1992) used another computer-digitiser system for measuring the distance in mm from implant shoulder to bone-implant contact mesially and distally. Reproducibility of repeated measurements reveals a standard deviation ($n = 8$) of 0.08-0.16 mm for one-stage non-submerged implants.

Ichikawa et al. (1990; 1994) used standardised radiography with a modified custom-made film holder to investigate the bone level around an apatite implant, which has a dense apatite outer tube and a titanium flanged inner tube (Apaceram, Pentax, Tokyo, Japan) (Ichikawa et al. 1990; 1994). The measurement error was expressed as the coefficient of variation (mean/SD), being 1.6% for the reproducibility of the radiographs and 0.6% for the accuracy of the measurements.

In general, the computerised determination of the bone level shows an improved detection of small bone level changes. On the other hand, some disadvantages of conventional intra-oral radiography remain unsolved:

- no information with respect to bone density
- only mesial and distal bone levels are evaluated

It has to be noted that for bone height assessment around endosseous implants, a digital sliding gauge is more easy to put into practice than a computerised image analysis (Meijer et al. 1993). In conclusion, it can be stated that detection of bone level changes of the order of 0.5 mm may be carried out using conventional radiographs in a strict paralleling technique. For detection of smaller changes, computerised methods and improved standardisation is needed. It should be mentioned that digital intra-oral radiography could become a good means to perform such computerised measurements in daily practice.

4.3
Peri-Implant Bone Height Changes

Radiography is usually not performed immediately after implant placement because of a fear that radiation would interfere with the healing (Brånemark et al. 1977). Indeed, there is a tendency for radiations to concentrate at a bone-metal interface by scattering (Carlsson 1973). Whether this is clinically relevant is unknown. In absence of early complications, the first radiograph of an installed two-stage implant is usually carried out at abutment connection (Fig. 4.14). During the first year of loading, a 12-month interval for radiographs can be recommended. Since rapid marginal bone loss is less frequently seen after the first year, the next follow-up radiograph could be made after two years, and then at 3 or 5-years intervals. The intervals between clinical visits remain however shorter (6m-1y), depending on the outcome of the clinical parameters of soft tissues.

For some two-stage implant systems, the mean marginal bone loss during the first year after abutment installation is between 0.5 to 1 mm, after which bone loss is limited to 0.05 mm to 0.1 mm per year (Adell et al. 1986; Quirynen et al. 1992a; Naert et al. 1992)(Fig. 4.15). One-stage non-submerged implants have a remodelling capacity of 0.59 – 1.09 mm during the first year. No significant bone changes seem to occur after the first year (Weber et al. 1992). It remains important to detect additional bone loss, which can be associated with implant surface characteristics (Pilliar et al. 1991), occlusal overload or persisting gingival inflammation (Quirynen et al. 1992b+c+d) (Fig. 4.16). It should be mentioned that not all commercially available implant systems fulfil the Albrektsson's success criteria. The latter also implies that the annual bone loss is higher than the aforementioned data. A number of oral implant systems are poorly documented or not followed for an adequate time period. Others that have been documented do not demonstrate acceptable success rates. Several authors reported a progressive marginal bone loss around IMZ plasma-sprayed implants (on average 0.5 mm/year even after 9 years (Malmqvist and Sennerby 1990; Richter et al. 1990; Schramm-Scherer et al. 1989; Quirynen et al. 1992a; Dietrich et al. 1993). Important marginal bone loss has also been reported around other roughened implant surfaces with increasing failure rates over time (Ledermann 1989; Block and Kent 1994; Versteegh et al. 1995). Using transmandibular implants in the edentulous mandible (TMI, Krijnen Medical BV, Beesd, The Netherlands), it has been stated that bone resorption can be arrested or that an increased bone apposition may occur (Powers et al. 1994). This observation should be interpreted cautiously, since bone height meas-

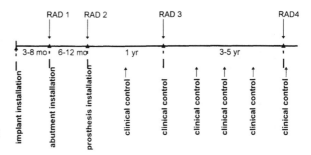

Fig. 4.14. Radiographic control scheme for implant follow-up

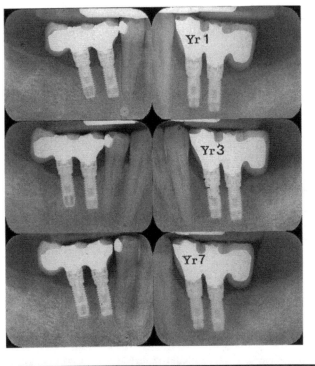

Fig. 4.15. Intra-oral radiographs of screw-shaped titanium implants followed during a 7-years period, showing a stabilisation of the bone loss after the first remodelling year

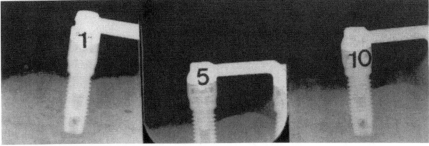

Fig. 4.16. Subsequent intra-oral radiographs of a screw-shaped titanium implant during a 10-years period, showing a substantial bone loss from year 1 to year 5 probably due to overloading. After correcting the load distribution, the bone level remained stable (year 10)

urements were carried out on panoramic radiographs, which are known to have a low diagnostic value, especially for linear measurements in the frontal area. Up till now, the Brånemark implant remains the only endosseous design with well-documented good long-term success rates.

It should be taken into account that the remodelling for the maxilla is much more important than for the mandible, so that mean remodelling rates cannot be extrapolated from one jaw to the other or from one site to another. Bone around one-stage non-submerged implants shows a different remodelling capacity for mandibular

(0.59 mm during the first year) and maxillary (1.09 mm during the first year) implants. The difference in remodelling capacity between maxilla and mandible is related to their different degree of vascularisation and bone density. Local bone quality has an important effect on this remodelling rate. Ahlqvist et al. (1990) claimed that there is a greater rate of marginal bone loss around implants in patients with initial minor jaw bone resorption compared to patient with initial advanced jaw bone resorption. Their observation was related to differences in remodelling capacity between different parts of the jaw bone. This observation merits further documentation, to allow definite conclusions.

Difficulties arise with regard to marginal bone measurements due to:

- variability in the radiographic process
- aids employed in interpretation
- perceptual ability of the observer

It should be noted that radiographic follow-up is costly and should be limited because of radiation risks. Besides, it only reveals the approximal areas. Attachment level measurements could therefore be considered as an alternative. The relationship between marginal bone level and attachment level as measured with a periodontal probe is well established (Quirynen et al. 1991b)(Fig. 4.17). The attachment level can be assessed as the sum of the periodontal pocket depth and the recession for each approximal site. The marginal bone level can be assessed as the distance between the top of the abutment or implant and the top of the bone in contact with the implant. When an intra-bony defect is present, one should only consider that part of the defect where a pocket probe could enter. This implies that one should calculate the corrected bone level, being the distance between the top of the abutment and the bone level

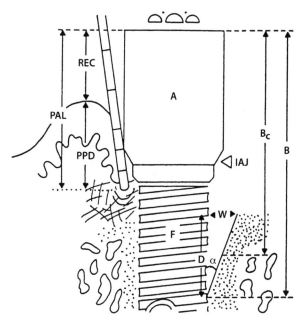

Fig. 4.17. Clinical and radiographic parameters to evaluate peri-implant tissues are schematically presented. F (= implant); A (= abutment), IAJ (= implant-abutment junction); REC (= recession): distance between marginal border of soft tissue and top of abutment; PPD (= pocket probing depth): distance between tip of pocket probe and marginal border of soft tissue; PAL (= probing attachment level): PAL = REC+PPD; B (= bone level): distance between top abutment and alveolar crest; W: width intra-bony defect; D: depth intra-bony defect; α: angle intra-bony defect; $D = W/tg(\alpha)$; B_c (= corrected bone level): $B_c = B-(0.5/tg(\alpha))$ (from Quirynen et al. 1991b)

where the width of the intra-bony defect is 0.5 mm or more (Quirynen et al. 1991b). The mean distance between the marginal bone level and the probing attachment level is, on average, between 1.2 and 1.4 mm, which corresponds to the connective tissue cuff observed around abutments (Van Drie et al. 1988). It is somewhat smaller than the distance mentioned for teeth (1.5 to 2.2 mm)(Van der Velden 1979).

Besides the peri-implant bone remodelling, the edentulous jaw bone more distant from the implants may also be influenced by the implant-supported prosthesis. Panoramic radiography was used for planimetrical evaluation of jaw bone changes in patients with fixed or removable implant-supported prostheses in the edentulous mandible (Jacobs et al. 1992; Jacobs et al. 1993). When evaluating bone resorption in the posterior mandible, significant bone resorption is noted for overdentures on 2 implants connected by a bar (Jacobs et al. 1992). For full fixed prostheses on 4-6 implants, jaw bone resorption is arrested. It should be mentioned that in either case, no significant bone resorption takes place after more than 10 years of edentulism. When evaluating maxillary bone resorption, significant bone resorption occurs in the anterior maxillary region for the implant-supported fixed prostheses but not for the overdentures (Jacobs et al. 1993). The increased anterior bone resorption could be compared to the Kelly phenomenon when only few mandibular front teeth are left. In either case, results indicate that relining and rebasing of the (over)denture should be carried out on a regular basis to preserve the correct vertical dimension.

When describing bony defects around cylindrical titanium implants on panoramic radiographs, it seems that such defects are usually found both mesially and distally, assuming that they circumscribe the entire neck of the implants (Mericske-Stern et al. 1994). This is not the case with other implants like the screw-shaped titanium implants (Lekholm et al. 1994).

Chapter 5

Bone Quality

5.1
Methodologies for Assessment of Alveolar Bone Quality

Besides quantitative information on the bone volume, radiographs may give a rough estimate of the bone quality besides indications of pathologic changes that could interfere with the subsequent implant treatment. The darkness of radiographical images depends on the light absorbing and scattering properties of the silver grains as well as on the fraction of radiation that is transmitted. The latter is related to the bone width and mineral content. When viewing a two-dimensional radiograph, information on bone width is evidently scarce. The superimposition of structures renders interpretation of a radiograph even more complex. Conventional intra-oral radiography does not reveal significant changes of the cancellous bone.

A loss of more than 30–50 % of trabecular bone is needed before radiographic detection occurs (Agus and Goldberg 1972; Shapiro 1972). While bone loss in the trabecular part is hardly detected, lesions extending through the trabeculo-cortical border are more prone to be detected (Van der Stelt 1985). Furthermore, a change in the trabecular pattern is only observed when the transitional trabeculo-cortical area is damaged.

The poor detection capacity of intra-oral radiographs is not only caused by variations in projection geometry and their two-dimensional nature, but also by the variations in contrast and density of the radiograph. The latter variations may be explained by uncontrolled film processing and variability in KVp and exposure time.

To assess bone and bone changes a three-dimensional technique is needed. A number of diagnostic techniques for bone density measurements of the different parts of the skeleton are currently available:

- photon absorptiometry (single/dual)
- x-ray absorptiometry (single/dual)
- quantitative computer tomography
- ultrasonography, ...

Each of these techniques may assess bone mass differently. These techniques are mostly not suitable for clinical evaluation of the jaw bone. von Wowern (1985) developed a dual photon absorptiometry apparatus for jaw bone mass measurements. A precision of 2.1% was reported *in vivo* (coefficient of variation = SD/mean; von Wowern et al. 1988). When applying this technique, it was possible to prove the relationship between mandibular bone mass and skeletal cortical but not trabecular bone mass (von Wowern et al. 1988). von Wowern and co-workers were the only research group to apply this technique, especially developed to monitor the jaw bone density.

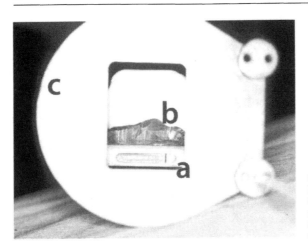

Fig. 5.1. Individualised bite block (a) including a calibrated aluminium wedge (b), to be radiographed with the intra-oral film using a beam-aiming device (c)

Other authors tried dual photon absorptiometry without further adaptation of the apparatus. The precision of such measurements by means of equipment which is calibrated and used for long bones can be questioned (Corten et al. 1993).

Other techniques for bone quality assessment of the jaw bones have been reported. Three-dimensional information can be gained from a two-dimensional radiograph by placing a calibrating wedge of a known composition and thickness on the film in a reproducible position in relation to the teeth and the radiation source (Fig. 5.1). Aluminium can be used as a reference material because it is homogeneous and easily machined and because the absorption and scatter properties are similar to those of bone (Trouerbach 1982). The bone structures are then radiographed together with this wedge. Such an aluminium wedge may produce the same optical density as in an

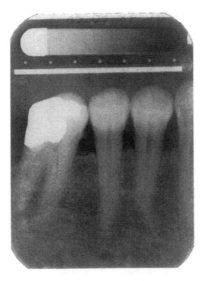

Fig. 5.2. The aluminium wedge produces the same optical density as in an area of interest on the radiograph

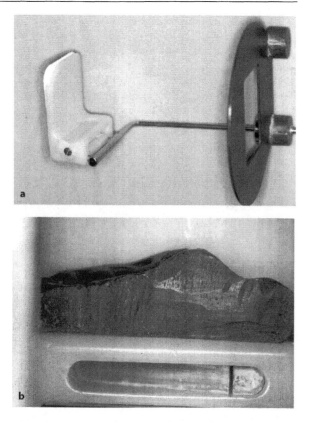

Fig. 5.3. Film holder with bite block **(a)** and individual stent **(b)** for standardised paralleling radiography of the region of interest

area of interest on the radiograph (Fig. 5.2). By scanning and digitising the radiograph, density curves are obtained for the aluminium wedge, which permit to calculate the Al thickness equivalent (Al eq value of bone) for each spot along the bone scan, showing the same absorption and thus the same blackening on the film. Digital subtraction radiography has increased the detection sensitivity of jaw bone density changes. It is based on the elimination of constant structures between two images, thus enhancing the structures demonstrating changes in density. Obtaining a doublet or a series of radiographs for digital subtraction implies a standardisation of projection geometry, exposure time and film processing procedure. A standardised projection geometry may be obtained by combining an individualised biteblock and a beam-aiming device (Duckworth et al. 1983; Pitts 1984; Harrison and Richardson 1989; Janssen et al. 1989; Baddock and Arnold 1990; Zappa et al. 1991), by reducing the angular discrepancy using a cephalostat and increasing the x-ray source to film distance (Jeffcoat et al. 1987) or by digitally correcting misangulation errors applying algorithms (Jeffcoat et al. 1984)(Fig. 5.3).

Absolute measurements of bone mineral change can be obtained from subtraction radiographs, in which anatomic structures that have not changed between examinations are displayed on a neutral background. A densitometric reference wedge is presented to avoid fluctuations in brightness and/or contrast of the radiographs and to provide a reference for bone mass (Vos et al. 1986; Brägger et al. 1987; Webber et al. 1990; Jeffcoat et al. 1992b; Jeffcoat and Reddy 1993). These wedges may be included in one (Jeffcoat et al. 1992b; Jeffcoat and Reddy 1993) or both of the images to be subtracted (Vos et al. 1986; Brägger et al. 1987; Webber et al. 1990; Galgut et al. 1991; Ichikawa et al. 1994; Jacobs et al. 1996). In contrast to absolute methods, relative methods do not use a reference wedge but express osseous changes by defined units of change in grey level (Strid 1985 a+b; Brägger 1988). Colour conversion of the grey

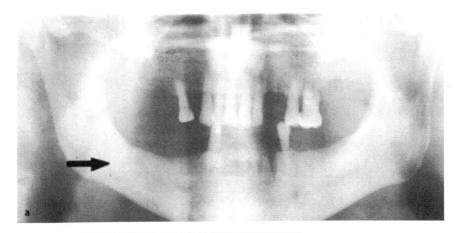

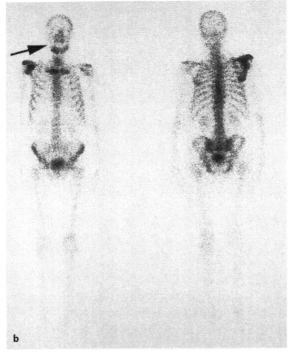

Fig. 5.4. a Panoramic radiograph of a patient showing an altered trabecular pattern on the right side of the mandible (arrow). b Technetium scintigraphy of the skeleton indicates that there is an abnormal resorption and apposition of osseous tissue on this side (arrow). Besides, the bladder is also found positive and a Paget's disease is diagnosed (from the Department of Radiology, University Hospital Gasthuisberg, Leuven, Belgium)

shades may facilitate the detection of bone loss (different colours for areas of bone loss or gain).

Apart from the aforementioned procedures, radioisotope scintigraphy using technetium-99m-methylene diphosphonate (Tc-99m-MDP) is a useful and reliable clinical method for measuring increased metabolic activity of the skeletal tissue (Stromqvist et al. 1987; Meidan et al. 1994)(Fig. 5.4). It could thus theoretically be applied for visualising peri-implant remodelling in the jaw bone. Two hours after injection of the isotope, the jaw may be scanned using a gamma-camera and the levels for isotope uptake are detected, stored and analysed by a computer. Since the absolute count is dependent on the individual bone mass, the time of administration and the rate of metabolism, the density count at the peri-implant tissue is expressed with reference to the skull or the surrounding jaw bone (Meidan et al. 1994).

5.2
Methodologies for Assessment of Peri-Implant Bone Quality

5.2.1
Conventional Intra-Oral Radiographs

To assess peri-implant bone quality on conventional radiographs, a classification of peri-implant bone quality was introduced by Adell et al. (1986):

Score 1 = cancellous trabecular bone along the entire implant contour
Score 2 = radiopaque zone marginally with cancellous trabecular bone surrounding the deeper part of the implant
Score 3 = radiopaque zone surrounding the implant entirely

Although this method has been capable of demonstrating an enhancement of radiopacity in the coronal part of an implant under functional loading, it remains a qualitative, non-objective attempt for bone density assessment. More objective and accurate methods were therefore developed. Strid (1985 a, b) applied computerised image analysis for photodensitometric scanning of peri-implant bone yields information regarding bone density changes. A density increase along the implant surface indicates an ongoing bone mineralisation, a density decrease or radiolucency surrounding the implant implies non-integration and implant failure. This allows to distinguish between real fibrous encapsulation and so-called Mach bands phenomenon (see § 4.2.1). Although this method is highly sensitive to quantify peri-implant bone density, only single scans can be evaluated. Digitalisation and storage of the entire image is not possible, but one can detect non-osseointegration or increased bone density around functionally loaded implants.

5.2.2
Digital Subtraction Radiography

The procedure of digital subtraction radiography has increased the sensitivity by which it is possible to detect bone density changes around implants. The application of digital subtraction radiography in the evaluation of peri-implant tissues has already been reported in animal research (Fourmousis et al. 1994a), case presentations (Engelke et al. 1990; Reddy et al. 1992; Jeffcoat et al. 1992a; Jeffcoat and Reddy 1993) or limited patient samples with apatite implants (Ichikawa et al. 1994). Digital subtraction radiography may be carried out in different ways. Some of the procedures are summarised below.

1. Standardised radiographs may be digitised using a black and white CCD camera, specially adapted for picture processing. Prior to subtraction of two standardised radiographs, superimposition is performed by interactively shifting and rotating the follow-up radiograph (Fourmousis et al. 1994b). The use of reference points in the images for digital superposition seems superior to this manual method (Wenzel 1989). Amalgam fillings or implants may be considered as optimal landmarks for the positioning of the reference points. Afterwards, density changes caused by difference in exposure and/or developing conditions may be corrected, by comparing and adjusting the 2 images. After subtraction, areas of interest can be identified on the baseline picture, allowing the evaluation of bone change in suspected areas.

2. Another procedure consists of using standardised radiography to investigate the bone level around an apatite implant with a dense apatite outer tube and a titanium flanged inner tube (e.g. Apaceram) (Ichikawa et al. 1990; 1994). Film contrast is corrected by comparing the contrast of copper steps (0.1-0.8 mm) placed on sequential x-ray films. Bone density changes are indicated using pseudo-coloured subtraction images, in which colour changes demonstrate a difference in density.

3. A third method was described by Jeffcoat et al. (1992b). After digitalisation and correction for contrast and planar geometric discrepancies, the first radiograph is subtracted from the second. The resultant subtraction image contains an aluminium reference wedge, which has only been presented in the first radiograph. The differences in grey level between baseline and follow-up image are expressed as changes in aluminium equivalent. The mass of the lesion is calculated by multiplying the area with the thickness and with the aluminium-to-bone density conversion factor. The calculated lesion size is not an absolute measure of the lesion mass, but may be reliable enough to express bone mass changes, even before these changes are clinically detectable. A good correlation has been established between the computed and actual "lesion" mass. Such correlation was also found by Webber et al. (1990). In an *in vitro* study using sections of pig mandible with hollow cylinder titanium implants, a bone change of 1 mg could be detected on conventionally exposed radiographs (0.44 s)(Fourmousis et al. 1994a). Underexposed radiographs (0.13 s) were able to recognise soft tissue specimens of 1 – 6 mg in an approximal defect (Fourmousis et al. 1994a).

Despite the increased sensitivity of these methods the interpretation of buccal and/or oral defects remains difficult because of the 2-dimensional nature of the radiograph. A bone mass change of at least 14 mg is needed to be detected by digital subtraction. The latter defects can also be detected with less demanding methods. This can be explained by the high radiographic density of the implant, which may saturate the buccal and/or oral space of the implant on the radiograph. The high radiographic density of the implant can also lead to the typical Mach bands (Ratliff 1965) which should be differentiated from the presence of a soft tissue space between implant and bone (Hollender 1992). Digital subtraction radiography allows this discrimination.

In conclusion, digital subtraction with high-quality, standardised radiographs may thus be used for:

- peri-implant radiolucency
- bone density measurements and changes around different implant materials in the jaw bone
- detection of peri-implant marginal bone level changes < 0.5 mm

This method is however not ready for routine clinical use. Its disadvantages are:

- exact superimposition of the radiographs is required (individual impression for reproducible film holder position)
- changes in occlusion may interfere with standardisation
- standardisation of all procedures involved in radiographic follow-up remains critical
- time-consuming and expensive
- information on bone, buccal and lingual of the implant is still lacking

Another method to evaluate bone remodelling around implants over time would be to digitise panoramic radiographs and examine a region of interest. The latter could be of interest to perform research in centres where panoramic radiographs are taken on a routine basis. On these radiographs, image texture is less susceptible to magnification and distortion and therefore, fractal analysis of the peri-implant bone may reveal information on bone remodelling (Wilding et al. 1995).

5.2.3
Digital Intra-Oral Radiography

Film-free radiology requires a sensor for detection, a computer memory for storage and a monitor for display. A number of techniques are currently available for clinical use (see chapter 1). Digital radiography enables storage, manipulation and correction of the image for under- and overexposures and allows a more reproducible and objective measurement.

For densitometric measurements, one may choose to display:

- a histogram, showing the distribution of the grey levels within the image (Fig. 5.5a)
- a line profile, measuring the grey levels on a selected line (Fig. 5.5b)
- a scaled profile, measuring the average density profiles along consecutive parallel lines within a selected area (Fig. 5.5c)

This may prove to be beneficial for detecting bone density changes over time. Density changes can also be easily visualised by colour enhancement. To obtain quantitative measurements of bone density changes, a standardised long cone paralleling technique is required. Digital radiography undergoes a rapid evolution and could become of great interest to evaluate peri-implant bone level and density changes.

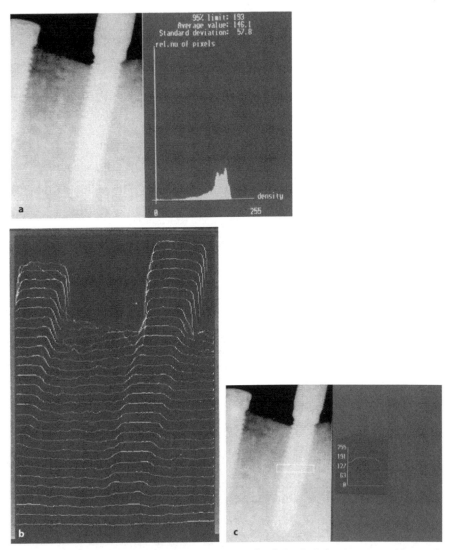

Fig. 5.5. Direct digital radiograph (Sens-a-ray, Regam, Sundsvall, Sweden) showing an osseointegrated screw-shaped implant. Densitometric analyses show a histogram of the grey levels (**a**), line profiles of grey levels (**b**) and a scaled profile within a selected area (**c**)

5.3
Peri-Implant bone density changes

In a longitudinal observation on screw-shaped titanium implants the bone-implant interface shows an increased density over the years (Strid 1985b). This is revealed by the increased slope on the horizontal density measurement line (line profile). This zone of increased density also seems to widen over the years. This observation has been confirmed by other authors (Fig. 5.6). von Wowern et al. (1990) reported an increased bone density over time around endosseous titanium implants supporting overdentures in the lower jaw. Wilding and co-workers (1995) could identify an increased bone density distally from the posterior implants of fixed implant-supported prostheses in the lower jaw. Ichikawa et al. (1994) observed an increased bone density around apatite implants especially in the crestal region, up to 2 years after implant installation.

It is interesting to report that the rigidity of the bone to implant interface also seems to increase over the years as revealed by decreased Periotest (Periotest, Siemens AG, Bernsheim, Germany) values. The latter are measurements expressed in arbitrary units as performed by an electronic device which delivers standardised taps by means of a rod projected against the abutment. It measures the resulting deceleration of the rod (Teerlinck et al. 1991; van Steenberghe et al. 1995). One does not need radiographs in clinical practice to measure the rigidity of the bone-implant continuum and the interface in particular since this non-invasive method also reveals the increase of its rigidity over time (Tricio et al. 1995). This kind of measurement can help the prosthodontist or restorative dentist to decide if the interface can already take important occlusal loads or if on the contrary the healing phase is far from ended. This might encourage him to wait before installing a fixed prosthesis with long cantilevers.

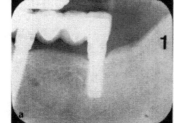
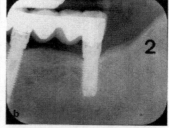
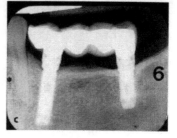

Fig. 5.6. A series of intra-oral radiographs indicating an increased bone density over a 5-years period of functional loading. **a** Examination at year 1 after the initial remodelling; **b** Examination at year 2 showing bone loss as a result of initial remodelling; **c** At year 6, an increased density of the peri-implant bone can be visually detected, especially around the distal implant

Lack of osseointegration refers to the interposition of fibrous tissue between the implant surface and the surrounding bone and is often reflected in clinical mobility and/or peri-implant radiolucency. Nevertheless, the sensitivity of both clinical parameters remains insufficient. With regard to implant mobility assessments, the use of an electronic device or determination of the damping characteristics of implants (Periotest) may offer a highly reproducible tool to detect subclinical mobilities. In the study by Teerlinck et al. (1991), 60 Brånemark mandibular implants were investigated. Repeated measurements indicated an accuracy of 1 Periotest value for 95% of the measurements. It was recently observed that the Periotest value decreased over a period of time (van Steenberghe et al. 1995), which parallels with the increased bone mineralisation noted at the interface (Strid 1985b; Johansson and Albrektsson 1987). The prognostic factor of this device could however not yet be assessed, due to the limited number of implant failures in the system concerned.

Digital subtraction radiography has also been used to detect implant failure. Jeffcoat et al. (1992a) reported that it was possible to visualise non-osseointegration of

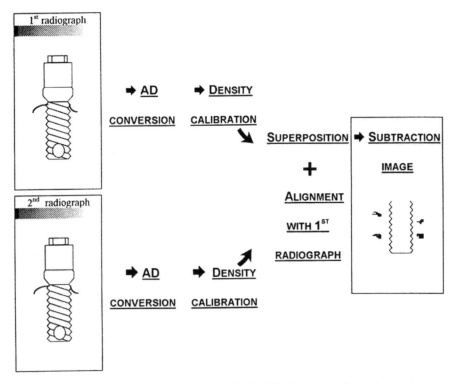

Fig. 5.7. Schematic presentation of one procedure for digital subtraction radiography (Jacobs et al. 1996), which could be used to evaluate the peri-implant bone density over time. The subtraction image only visualises the regions of bone density change. It could yield an increasing density for functionally loaded implants or a decreasing density for failing implants

an implant after 3 months, whereas the clinical measure of increased mobility could only be established after 9 months. The ability of this technique to detect clinically non-integrated implants claims a 100 % sensitivity and specificity (Jeffcoat and Reddy 1993) (Fig. 5.7).

Chapter 6

Radiographic Assessment of Implant Complications and/or Failures

6.1
Introduction

Endosseous implants offer a predictable prognosis even over decades when they are properly osseointegrated. This term has been coined by P-I Brånemark and has corresponded to several definitions over time. The concept is, that after an intimate bone-to-implant surface contact has been established, a stable interface is created withstanding the challenges of load and oral microbiota for decades. Since then, the term has been adopted by many, and often misused, limiting it to the intimate bone-to-implant contact. The latter can be achieved by many different implant surfaces, although several, especially some with a roughened surface texture, exhibit progressive marginal bone loss over the years. The latter breakdown is not compatible with the implications of the osseointegration concept.

In clinical practice, it is of extreme importance to find out whether an intimate bone-to-implant contact has been achieved, and afterwards whether the marginal bone level remains stable over time. Thus, two general principles must be kept in mind to make radiographic diagnosis useful:

- definition
- repeated observations

6.2
Assessment of Bone-to-Implant Interface

Since even intra-oral radiographs taken with a paralleling technique have no discrimination power below 0.2 mm (Benn 1992), one cannot expect them to confirm a histological state. On the other hand if a continuous radiolucency appears at the implant-bone interface (Fig. 6.1a), one can clearly state that the implant is surrounded by a non-mineralised (probably scar) tissue (Sundén and Gröndahl 1995). Thus, the radiographic diagnosis is a negative one, i.e. absence of bone apposition. It has been observed that such fibrously encapsulated implants are prone to surinfections of the peri-implant pockets, similar to what is observed in periodontitis (Fig. 6.1b–d). Therefore, most clinicians prefer to remove such implants as soon as possible before important bone cratering occurs. In a severely resorbed mandible such cratering presents risks for osteomyelitis and jaw bone fracture (Fig. 6.2).

One should be aware of the optic phenomenon, called the Mach bands effect (see § 4.2), frequently occurring around implants (Hollender 1992). It is not always easy to distinguish between a true radiolucency and this optic phenomenon. Therefore, this

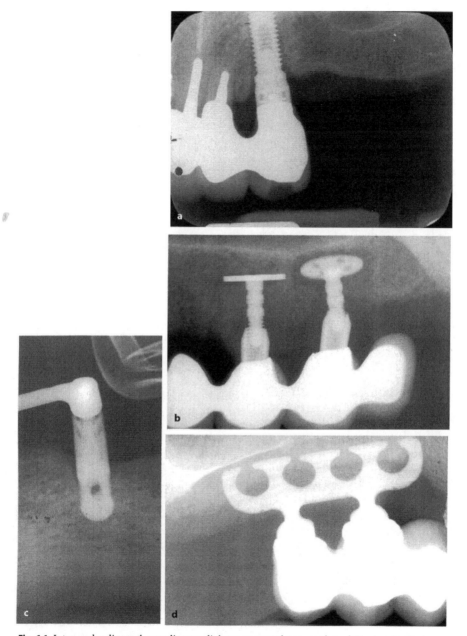

Fig. 6.1. Intra-oral radiograph revealing a radiolucency around a screw-shaped titanium implant, confirming the clinical signs of non-osseointegration (**a**). Other radiographs show fibrously encapsulated implants, which have been surinfected: **b** disk-form **c** cylindric, **d** blade-form

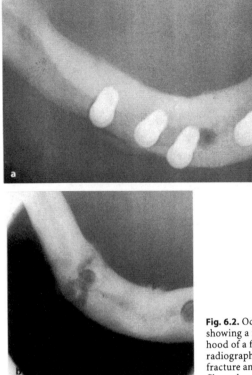

Fig. 6.2. Occlusal radiograph of an edentulous patient showing a fracture of the mandible in the neighbourhood of a fibrously encapsulated implant **(a)**. Occlusal radiograph of another patient showing a mandibular fracture and osteomyelitis after removal of surinfected fibrously encapsulated implants **(b)**

radiographic diagnosis should be in agreement with clinical mobility and/or rigidity (Periotest) diagnosis. If there is no agreement, one should have a second look at the radiograph.

At the so-called "apical" end of implants a small round radiolucency can sometimes be observed. This can be the result of the drilling procedure which went deeper than the implant length (Fig. 6.3). This is a regular uneventful happening. It takes some time before this alveolus is remineralised. Overheating can also lead to a reaction around the tip of the implant, which can reveal itself as a radiolucency (Fig. 6.4). This should be differentiated from the presence of the mental foramen in the neighbourhood of the implant (Fig. 6.5).

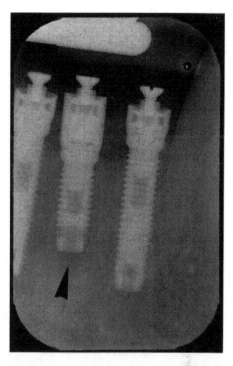

Fig. 6.3. Intra-oral radiograph revealing a small round radiolucency of a recently installed screw-shaped titanium implant, as a result of the drilling procedure (arrow)

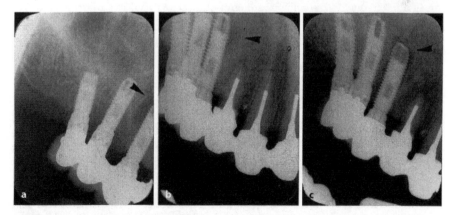

Fig. 6.4. Intra-oral radiographs of a screw-shaped titanium implant with a peri-apical radiolucency (arrow). It was assumed that this was caused by overheating during the drilling procedure (**a:** year *1*). The defect diminished after removal of the fibrogranulomatous tissue at year *4* (**b**) and almost disappeared after a second surgical procedure at year *6* (**c**)

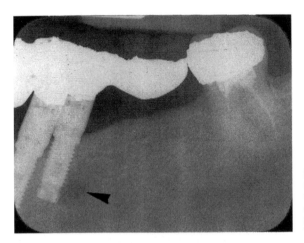

Fig. 6.5. The radiolucency (arrow) in the neighbourhood of the implant is caused by overlapping of the mental foramen and the implant on the two-dimensional radiograph

Finally, the stress concentrations around loaded implants occur, according to the finite element analysis mathematical models, at the marginal bone level and around the implant tip. At the marginal bone level this leads more or less systematically to a limited angular defect (see § 6.3) while at the tip of the implant this is rarely visible. Indeed, it is known from studies on dry skulls, that as long as lesions remain confined to the cancellous bone they remain radiographically invisible, while the slightest cortical lesion appears at once (Van der Stelt 1985). It is plausible that such lesions occur much more frequently but remain radiographically silent, unless a CT scan would be taken after implant installation. This is hardly ever useful.

6.3
Assessment of Marginal Bone Level Stability

As has been discussed in the preceding paragraph, after loading, most implant configurations lead to a stress concentration at the marginal bone level which reveals itself on intra-oral radiographs as small (some 1 mm) angular bony defects (Fig. 6.6). This is observed during the first months after occlusal loading (Hoshaw et al. 1994). Some have argued that this would be the result of the countersinking which is advocated by a number of implant systems during implant installation. The idea of countersinking is to widen the entrance of the drilled alveolus to increase the contact surface of the "shoulder" of the implant and the cortical bone. This hypothesis has been proven to be wrong since with implant configurations which do not apply a countersink procedure (e.g. the 5 mm diameter implant of the Brånemark system) the same bony angular defects appear after loading (see Fig. 6.6). Others, still refuting the evidence of stress concentration, associated these defects with a soft tissue inflammation which would result from the leakage of bacteria from the interstitium between implants and abutment. It is true that such leakage has been observed (Quirynen et al. 1993) but the relationship with bone loss was never put forward by those that reported it. The same kind of screw-shaped titanium implants are in use in hand surgery, where they are installed in the metacarpal bones and proximal phalanges. Here

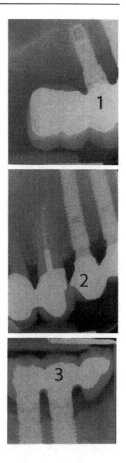

Fig. 6.6. Intra-oral radiograph of screw-shaped titanium implants show-ing small angular defects around the neck of the implant as a result of stress concentration after loading, with (1) or without (2, 3) using a countersinking procedure:

1. Brånemark system screw-shaped implants (3.75 mm ø)

2. Astra screw-shaped implants (3.5 mm ø)

3. Brånemark system screw-shaped implants (5.0 mm ø)

too, where evidently no bacteria or plaque is present, angular defects appear soon after loading (Lundborg 1996 personal communication).

Another argument is the clinical observation of deeper defects when excessive occlusal loads are present (Fig. 6.7). In these instances, the bone loss can reach several millimeters, but finally stabilises, or even seems radiographically reversible. One can conclude with little doubt that the small angular defects which appear at the marginal bone within the first year after occlusal loading are associated with stress concentra-tions. After this early fast remodelling period, the bone level tends to stabilise or a minimal loss is observed (0.05 mm/year for the Brånemark system)(Fig. 6.8). Not only stress concentration but also stress shielding may cause bone loss. Screw-shaped implants with a smooth conical upper third show indeed bone loss up to the first implant thread (Quirynen et al. 1992c) (Fig. 6.9).

For a number of implant configurations on the other hand, a clinically significant ongoing marginal bone loss has been observed radiographically. A well-documented example is the titanium plasma-sprayed cylindrical implant (IMZ) where no less than 6 different centres reported an annual marginal bone loss of 0.4 to 0.6 mm which does

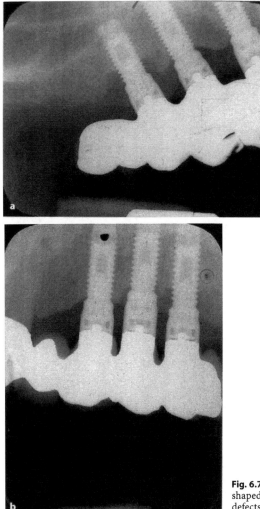

Fig. 6.7. Intra-oral radiographs of screw-shaped titanium implants with deeper angular defects caused by excessive occlusal loads related to bruxism

not seem to stabilise even after 4 to 6 years of observation (Malmqvist and Sennerby 1990; Richter et al. 1990; Schramm-Scherer et al. 1989; Quirynen et al. 1992a; Dietrich et al. 1993) (Fig. 6.10). The same ongoing loss of bone has been observed around other roughened surfaces (plasma-sprayed or coated with calcium-phosphates) (Ledermann 1989; Block and Kent 1994; Versteegh et al. 1995).

It is difficult to determine the cause of such ongoing bone loss. It is evident that all those surfaces revealed histologically in animal experiments an intimate implant-to-bone contact after insertion. This seems to indicate (see § 6.2) that the latter interface is not sufficient in se to claim osseointegration. This is even more true for bone apposition at the radiographic level. A possible explanation for the bone loss observed

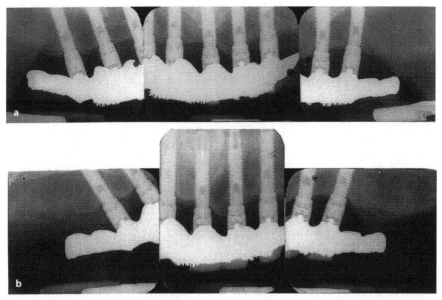

Fig. 6.8. A series of intra-oral radiographs of an edentulous patient, who was rehabilitated by means of 6 osseointegrated implants supporting a full fixed prosthesis in the upper jaw. After the first remodelling year, the bone level remained stable during the following years. **a** year 1; **b** year 11

around these types of implants is an intense soft tissue inflammatory reaction, triggered by gross plaque accumulation on the rough surface. A number of authors have hypothesised that something like peri-implantitis exists, by which they mean a plaque-induced inflammatory reaction similar to what occurs in periodontitis. Arguments have been collected from animal experiments where a ligature-induced acute inflammatory reaction around implants in beagle dogs seems to lead to a self-perpetuating marginal bone loss even around machined (i.e. only slightly roughened) implant surfaces (Lindhe et al. 1992). Clinically this has not been observed with the latter type of implant surfaces (Adell et al. 1986; Lekholm et al. 1986; van Steenberghe et al. 1993), so the question remains open.

Table 6.1. Preferred radiographic imaging procedures for pre-operative treatment planning and post-operative follow-up of oral implants

	Time (months)	Radiographic procedures
Treatment planning		
• screening	?	intra-oral, panoramic
• implant placement	−1	CT, panoramic, intra-oral
Implant placement	0	no radiograph, exc. problems
Healing period	0–4(6)	no radiograph, exc. problems
Remodelling period	4(6)–12	parallel long-cone radiography
Maintenance	+13	
• no clinical problems	Yr 3, 5, 10	parallel long-cone radiography
• clinical problems	any time	parallel long-cone radiography

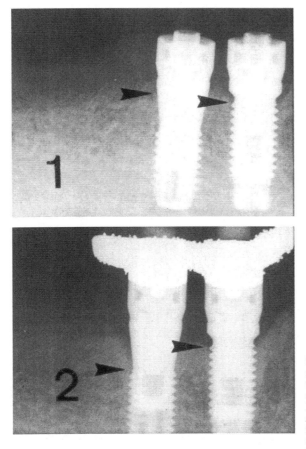

Fig. 6.9. Long-cone parallel radiographs of screw-shaped titanium implants at abutment surgery (1) and 1 year later (2). During this follow-up (from 1 to 2), bone loss occurred up to the first thread around the conical smooth part of the implant at the left side

Meanwhile it is of great clinical importance to find out in due time whether marginal bone loss occurs after the first year of intense bone remodelling at the marginal bone level. Indeed, since ongoing bone loss can be associated with mucosal inflammation or occlusal overload, measures can eventually be taken accordingly to limit or stop the process. Therefore preventive controls consist of intra-oral radiographs using a paralleling technique and an individual bite-block if the implant has not a threaded surface, at abutment installation (if a two-stage implant) and 1, 3, 5 and 10 years after prosthesis installation (Table 6.1). If some increased bone loss or other symptoms are observed more frequent exposures can be considered (Fig. 6.11). A threaded surface allows to check easily if a strict paralleling technique has been used; otherwise some blurring of the threads appears. The equal distances in between two threads (for example 0.6 mm) allows detection thresholds of 0.3 mm, which is unheard of around teeth. With a cylindrical design it is more difficult to detect changes in bone level (Sewerin 1991b). The use of subtraction radiography, so far more for experimental reasons, will soon become a clinical tool (Brägger et al. 1992).

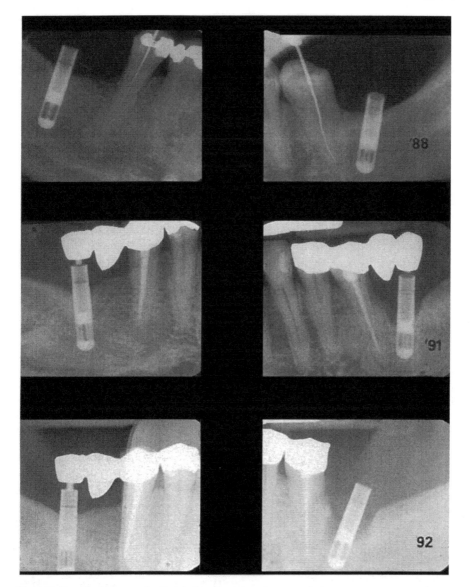

Fig. 6.10. Two plasma-sprayed cylindrical implants have been installed in the mandibular premolar regions. Over a 4-years period, the implant in the third quadrant has lost an important amount of bone

A drawback of radiographs is that they can only reveal bone loss at the mesial and distal sides of the implants, while due to the anatomy of the jaw bone, dehiscences and fenestration rather occur labially and orally. The latter can be prone to further bone loss and will remain unnoticed, because of the superimposition of the radiopaque implant body. Since for a screw-shaped implant – extrapolation should be confirmed

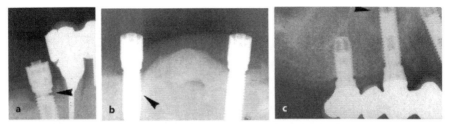

Fig. 6.11. Intra-oral radiographs are sometimes essential to help making a diagnosis for the patient's complaints. **a** fracture of a screw-shaped implant (arrow), **b** non-osseointegration of a screw-shaped implant (arrow), **c** peri-"apical" radiolucency around a screw-shaped implant (arrow)

by experimental evidence – it has been shown that probing attachment and marginal bone levels correlate highly (van Steenberghe and Quirynen 1993), this type of measurements should complement and sometimes replace radiographic controls. The absolute difference between the two is on average 1.5 mm, which means that the tip of the probe is stopped by the cuff of connective tissue some 1.5 mm coronally of the bone.

Some success criteria include marginal bone level measurements. This has led to the terminology of "failing" implants, which refers to an implant still in place and still functional but where ongoing marginal bone loss is observed. The very different radiographic criteria used in literature render comparisons often without meaning.

6.4
CT-Scan Images

The use of CT-scan to check the integration of an implant into the bone is not useful, since the discrimination power is too limited. Furthermore, the scatter that always results at the interface, because of reflection of the x-rays by the more impenetrable implant surface, renders interpretation of pictures even more hazardous. One of the possible indications for the use of CT scans to examine implants when complications occur is after the maxillary sinus or the mandibular canal have been penetrated. For the latter, when observed a few days after surgery, for example when the patient reports numbness of the lower lip, it can lead to a slight or complete removal of the responsible implant. When it relates to sinus penetration, a common uneventful happening, it can allow the surgeon to prove that the mucosal pathology was already existing before implant installation.

Summary

Placement of oral endosseous implants has become a common method of treatment for both completely and partially edentulous patients. A careful pre-operative radiographic examination remains a prerequisite for optimal installation of implants from a surgical as well as from a prosthetic point of view. Interference with certain anatomic structures may cause serious problems for the patient, such as loss of the implant or paraesthesiae. Intra-oral radiography has been used for many years as a routine examination of specific regions of the jaw bones. To more precisely determine jaw bone quality and quantity for pre-operative planning for implant rehabilitation, specialised radiological examinations have to be carried out. CT scanning remains the method of choice for pre-operative planning and implant placement in maxillary and distal mandibular areas. Besides the pre-operative radiographic planning, a radiographic follow-up of endosseous implants is required to evaluate the peri-implant bone remodelling and possibly detect complications. For the radiological follow-up, standardised radiographs are needed. Optimally, an intra-oral digital radiograph taken with the long-cone paralleling technique may reveal precise quantitative information of the peri-implant bone. Digitalisation and subtraction may objectivate the bone density.

References

Abrahams JJ (1993) Anatomy of the jaws revisited with a Dental CT software program. Amer J Neuroradiol 14: 979–990

Adell R, Lekholm U, Rockler B, Brånemark P-I (1981) A 15-years study of osseointegrated implants in the treatment of the edentulous jaw. Int J Oral Surg 10: 387–416

Adell R, Eriksson B, Lekholm U, Brånemark P-I, Jemt T (1990) A long-term follow-up study of osseointegrated implants in the treatment of totally edentulous jaws. Int J Oral Maxillofac Implants 5: 347–359

Adell R (1992) The surgical principles of osseointegration. In: Worthington P, Brånemark P-I, eds. Advanced osseointegration surgery. Applications in the maxillofacial region. Chicago: Quintessence Publ Co Inc, pp.94–107

Adell R, Lekholm U, Rockler B, Brånemark P-I, Lindhe J, Eriksson B, Sbordone L (1986) Marginal tissue reactions at osseointegrated titanium fixtures (I). A 3-year longitudinal prospective study. Int J Oral Maxillofac Surg 15: 39–52

Agus ZS, Goldberg M (1972) Pathogenesis of uremic osteodystrophy. Radiol Clin North Am 10: 545–556

Ahlqvist J, Borg K, Gunne J, Nilson H, Olsson M, Åstrand P (1990) Osseointegrated implants in edentulous jaws: A 2-year longitudinal study. Int J Oral Maxillofac Implants 5: 155–163

Albrektsson T, Jacobsson M (1987) Bone-metal interface in osseointegration. J Prosthet Dent 57: 597–607

Albrektsson T, Zarb G (1993) Current interpretations of the osseointegrated response: clinical significance. Int J Prosthodont 6: 95–105

Albrektsson T, Bergman B, Folmer T, Henry P, Higuchi K, Klineberg I, Laney WR, Lekholm U, Oikarinen V, van Steenberghe D, Triplett RG, Worthington P, Zarb G (1988) A multicenter report on osseointegrated oral implants. J Prosthet Dent 60: 75–84

Albrektsson T, Zarb G, Worthington P, Eriksson AR (1986) The long-term efficacy of currently used dental implants: a review and proposed criteria of success. Int J Oral Maxillofac Implants 1: 11–25

Andersson JE, Svartz K (1988) CT-scanning in the preoperative planning of osseointegrated implants in the maxilla. Int J Oral Maxillofac Surg 17: 33–35

Andersson L, Kurol M (1987) CT scan prior to installation of osseointegrated implants in the maxilla. Int J Oral Maxillofac Surg 16: 50–55

Atwood DA (1962) Some clinical factors related to rate of resorption of residual ridges. J Prosthet Dent 12: 441–450

Baddock C, Arnold MT (1990) Film cassette for quality assurance of dental x-ray tubes. Br J Radiol 63: 720–722

Baumrind S, Ben-Bassat Y, Korm EL, Bravo LA, Curry S (1992) Mandibular remodeling measured on cephalograms: 2. a comparison of information from implant and anatomic best-fit superimpositions. Am J Orthod Dentofacial Orthop 102: 227–238

Becker W, Dahlin C, Becker BE, Lekholm U, van Steenberghe D, Higuchi K, Kultje C (1994) The use of e-PTFE barrier membranes for bone promotion around titanium implants placed into extraction sockets: a prospective multicenter study. Int J Oral Maxillofac Implants 9: 31–40

Benn DK (1992) Estimating the validity of radiographic measurements of marginal bone height changes around osseointegrated implants. Implant Dent 1: 79–83

Block MS, Kent JN (1994) Long-term follow-up on hydroxyapatite-coated cylindrical dental implants. J Oral Maxillofac Surg 52: 937–942

Bonnier L, Ayadi K, Vasdev A, Crouzet G, Raphael B (1991) Three-dimensional reconstruction in routine computerized tomography of the skull and the spine. J Neuroradiol 18: 250–266

Borg E, Gröndahl HG (1996) On the dynamic range of different X-ray photon detectors in intra-oral radiography. A comparison of image quality in film, charge-coupled device and storage phosphor systems. Dentomaxillofac Radiol 2: 82–88

Borrow JW, Smith JP (1996) Stent marker materials for computerised tomograph-assisted implant planning. Int J Periodontics Restorative Dent 16: 61–67

Brägger U (1988) Digital imaging in periodontal radiography. A review. J Clin Periodontol 15: 551–557

Brägger U (1994) Radiographic parameters for the evaluation of peri-implant tissues. Periodontology 2000 4: 87–97

Brägger U, Burgin W, Fourmoussis I, Lang NP (1992) Image processing for the evaluation of dental implants. Dentomaxillofac Radiol 21: 208–212

Brägger U, Litch J, Pasquali L, Kornman KS (1987) Computer assisted densitometric image analysis for the quantitation of radiographic alveolar bone changes. J Periodont Res 22: 227–229

Brånemark P-I , Hansson B-O, Adell R, Breine U, Lindström J, Hallén O, Ohman A (1977) Osseointegrated implants in the treatment of the edentulous jaw. Experience from a 10-year period. Scand J Plast Reconstr Surg 11(Suppl 16): 1–132

Brånemark P-I, Svensson B, van Steenberghe D (1995) Ten-years survival rates of fixed prostheses on four or six implants ad modum Brånemark in full edentulism. Clin Oral Impl Res 6: 227–231

Carlsson GA (1973) Dosimetry at interfaces: theoretical analysis and measurements by means of thermoluminescent LiF at plane interface between a low z-material and Al, Cu, Sn, Pb irradiated with 100 to 200 kV roentgen radiation. Acta Radiol Suppl Stockh 332: 1–64

Chaytor DV (1993) Clinical criteria for determining implant success: Bone. Int J Prosthodont 6: 145–152

Corten FGA, van 't Hof MA, Buijs WCAM, Hoppenbrouwers P, Kalk W, Corstens FHM (1993) Measurements of mandibular bone density ex vivo and in vivo by dual-energy x-ray absorptiometry. Arch Oral Biol 38: 215–219

Cox JF, Pharoah M (1986) An alternative holder for radiographic evaluation of tissue-integrated prostheses. J Prosthet Dent 56: 338–341

Dao TTT, Anderson JD, Zarb GA (1993) Is osteoporosis a risk factor for osseointegration of dental implants. Int J Oral Maxillofac Implants 8: 137–144

De Laat A, Horvath M, Bossuyt M, Fossion E, Baert AL (1993) Myogenous or arthrogenous limitation of mouth opening: correlations between clinical findings, MRI and clinical outcome. J Orofacial Pain 7: 150–155

Dietrich U, Lippold R, Dirmeier T, Behneke N, Wagner W (1993) Statistical results for making an implant prognosis, based on 2017 IMZ implants with various indications placed during the past 13 years. Z Zahnärztl Implantol IX: 9–18

Duckmanton NA, Austin BW, Lechner SK, Klineberg IJ (1994) Imaging for predictable maxillary implants. Int J Prosthodont 7: 77–80

Duckworth JE, Judy PF, Goodson JM, Socransky SS (1983) A method for geometric and densitometric standardization of intraoral radiographs. J Periodontol 54: 435–440

Dula K, Mini R, Van der Stelt PF, Lambrecht JT, Schneeberger P, Buser D (1996) Hypothetical mortality risk associated with spiral computed tomography of the maxilla and mandible. Eur J Oral Sci 104: 503–510

Eggen S (1969) Standardiserad intraoral röntgenteknik. Sveriges Tändläkarförb Tidning 61: 867–872

Eggen S (1976) Pre-marked dental X-ray measuring film for paralleling technique. Quintessence Int 10: 67–70

Ekestubbe A, Thilander A, Gröndahl H-G (1992) Absorbed doses and energy imparted from tomography for dental implant installation. Spiral tomography using the Scanora technique compared with hypocycloidal tomography. Dentomaxillofac Radiol 21: 65–69

Ekestubbe A, Gröndahl H-G (1993) Reliability of spiral tomography with the Scanora technique for dental implant planning. Clin Oral Impl Res 4: 195–202

el Charkawi HG (1989) Residual ridge changes under titanium plasma-sprayed screw implant systems. J Prosthet Dent 62: 576–580

Ellis DS, Toth B, Stewart WB (1992) Three dimensional imaging and computer-designed prostheses in the evaluation and management of orbitocranial deformities. Adv Ophthalmic Plast Reconstr Surg 9: 261–272

Engelke W, De Valk S, Ruttiman U (1990) The diagnostic value of subtraction radiography in the assessment of granular hydroxylapatite implants. Oral Surg Oral Med Oral Pathol 9: 636–641

Feine JS, de Grandmont P, Boudrias P, Brien N, LaMarche C, Taché R, Lund JP (1994a) Within-subject comparisons of implant-supported mandibular prostheses: Choice of prosthesis. J Dent Res 73: 1105–1111

Feine JS, Maskawi K, de Grandmont P, Donohue WB, Tanguay R, Lund JP (1994b) Within-subject comparisons of implant-supported mandibular prostheses: Evaluation of masticatory function. J Dent Res 73: 1646–1656

Fourmousis I, Brägger U, Bürgin W, Tonetti M, Lang NP (1994a) Digital image processing. II. In vitro quantitative evaluation of soft and hard peri-implant tissue changes. Clin Oral Impl Res 5: 105–114

Fourmousis I, Brägger U, Bürgin W, Tonetti M, Lang NP (1994b) Digital image processing. I Evaluation of gray level correction methods in vitro. Clin Oral Impl Res 5: 37–47

Frederiksen NL (1995) Diagnostic imaging in dental implantology. Oral Surg Oral Med Oral Pathol Oral Radiol Endod 80: 540–554

Frederiksen NL, Benson BW, Sokolowski TW (1994) Effective dose and risk assessment from film tomography used for dental implant diagnostics. Dentomaxillofac Radiol 23: 123–127

Frederiksen NL, Benson BW, Sokolowski TW (1995) Effective dose and risk assessment from computed tomography of the maxillofacial complex. Dentomaxillofac Radiol 24: 55–58

Fredholm U, Bolin A, Henrikson CO, Cederlund T (1994) Preoperative radiographic evaluation of implant sites by computed tomography. Swed Dent J 18: 213–219

Friberg B, Sennerby L, Roos J, Lekholm U (1995) Identification of bone quality in conjunction with insertion of titanium implants. Clin Oral Impl Res 6: 213–219

Fritz ME (1996) Implant therapy II. World Workshop in Periodontics. Annals Periodontol 1: 796–815

Galgut PN, Verrier J, Waite IM, Linney A, Cornick DE (1991) Computerized densitometric analysis of interproximal bone levels in a controlled clinical study into the treatment of periodontal bone defects with ceramic hydroxyapatite implant material. J Periodontol 62: 44–50

Ghyselen J, Vervliet E, van Steenberghe D (1987) Technieken voor kaakbotmetingen in de parodontologie. J Head Neck Pathol 6: 30–40

Granström G (1992) The use of hyperbaric oxygen to prevent implant loss in the irradiated patient. In: Worthington P, Brånemark P-I, eds. Advanced osseointegration surgery. Applications in the maxillofacial region. Chicago: Quintessence Publ Co Inc, pp 336–345

Grevers G, Assal J, Vogl T, Wilimzig C (1991) Three-dimensional magnetic resonance imaging in skull base lesions. Am J Otolaryngol 12: 139–145

Hansson LG, Eriksson L, Westesson PL (1992) Magnetic resonance evaluation after temporomandibular joint diskectomy. Oral Surg 1974: 801–810

Harrison R, Richardson D (1989) Bitewing radiographs of children taken with and without a film-holding device. Dentomaxillofac Radiol 18: 97–99

Heffez L, Mafee MF, Vaiana J (1988) The role of magnetic resonance imaging in the diagnosis and management of ameloblastoma. Oral Surg 65: 2–12

Heiken JP, Brink JA, Vannier MW (1993) Spiral (Helical) CT. Radiology 189: 647–656

Hollender L (1992) Radiographic examination of endosseous implants in the jaws. In: Worthington P, Brånemark P-I, eds. Advanced osseointegration surgery. Applications in the maxillofacial region. Chicago: Quintessence Publ Co Inc, pp 80–93

Hollender L, Rönnerman A, Thilander B (1980) Root resorption, marginal bone support and clinical crown length in orthodontically treated patients. Eur J Orthodont 2: 197–205

Hollender L, Rockler B (1980) Radiographic evaluation of osseointegrated implants of the jaws. Dentomaxillofac Radiol 9: 91–95

Hoshaw S, Brunski J, Cochran G (1994) Mechanical loading of Brånemark implants affects interfacial bone modeling and remodeling. Int J Oral Maxillofac Implants 9: 345–360

Ichikawa T, Horiuchi M, Miyamoto M, Horisaka Y (1990) Radiographic analysis of a two-piece apatite implant. Part I. Standardized radiographs and digital image processing. Int J Oral Maxillofac Implants 6: 63–69

Ichikawa T, Miyamoto M, Horisaka Y, Horiuchi M (1994) Radiographic analysis of a two-piece apatite implant. Part II. Preliminary report of 2-year observation. Int J Oral Maxillofac Implants 9: 214–222

Ismail YH, Azarbal M, Kapa SF (1995) Conventional linear tomography: protocol for assessing endosseous implant sites. J Prosthet Dent 73: 153–157

Jacobs R, Schotte A, van Steenberghe D, Quirynen M, Naert I (1992) Posterior jaw bone resorption in osseointegrated implant-supported overdentures. Clin Oral Impl Res 3: 63–70

Jacobs R, van Steenberghe D, Nys M, Naert I (1993) Maxillary bone resorption in patients with mandibular implant-supported overdentures or fixed prostheses. J Prosthet Dent 70: 135–140

Jacobs R, Ghyselen J, Koninckx P, van Steenberghe D (1996) Long-term bone mass evaluation of mandible and lumbar spine in a group of women receiving hormone replacement therapy. Eur J Oral Sci 104: 10–16

Jaffin R, Berman C (1991) The excessive loss of Brånemark fixtures in type IV bone: a 5-year analysis. J Periodontol 62: 2–4

Janssen PTM, van Palenstijn-Heldermann WH, Van Aken J (1989) The effect of in-vivo occurring errors in reproducibility of radiographs on the use of the subtraction technique. J Clin Periodontol 16: 53–58

Jeffcoat MK (1992a) Digital radiology for implant treatment planning and evaluation. Dentomaxillofac Radiol 21: 203–207

Jeffcoat MK (1992b) Radiographic methods for the detection of progressive alveolar bone loss. J Periodont Res 19: 434–440

Jeffcoat MK, Jeffcoat R, Williams RC (1984) A new method of the comparison of bone loss measurements on non-standardized radiographs. J Periodont Res 19: 434–440

Jeffcoat MK, Williams RC (1984) Relationship between linear and area measurements of radiographic bone levels using simple computerized techniques. J Periodont Res 19: 191–198

Jeffcoat MK, Reddy MS (1993) Digital subtraction radiography for longitudinal assessments of peri-implant bone change: method and validation. Adv Dent Res 7: 196–201

Jeffcoat MK, Reddy MS, van den Berg HR, Bertens E (1992) Quantitative digital subtraction radiography for the assessments of peri-implant bone change. Clin Oral Impl Res 3: 22–27

Jeffcoat MK, Reddy MS, Webber RL, Williams RC, Rüttiman UE (1987) Extraoral control of geometry for digital subtraction radiography. J Periodont Res 22: 392–402

Jemt T, Chai J, Harnett J, Heath MR, Hutton JE, Johns RB, McKenna S, McNamara DC, van Steenberghe D, Taylor R, Watson RM, Herrmann I (1996) A 5-year prospective multicenter follow-up report on overdentures supported by osseointegrated implants. Int J Oral Maxillofac Implants 11: 291–298

Johansson C, Albrektsson T (1987) Integration of screw implants in the rabbit: a 1-year follow-up of removal torque of titanium implants. Int J Oral Maxillofac Implants 2: 69–75

Johansson P, Strid K-G (1994) Assessment of bone quality from cutting resistance during implant surgery. Int J Oral Maxillofac Implants 9: 279–288

Karellos ND, Zouras CS (1993) Transfer of CT scan data to diagnostic casts. Implant Dent 2: 97–99

Kassebaum DK, Stoller NE, McDavid WD, Goshorn B, Ahrens CR (1992) Absorbed dose determination for tomographic implant site assessment techniques. Oral Surg Oral Med Oral Pathol 73: 502–509

Klein HM, Schneider W, Alzen G, Voy ED, Günther RW (1992) Pediatric craniofacial surgery: comparison of milling and stereolithography for 3D model manufacturing. Pediatr Radiol 22: 458–460

Klinge B, Petersson A, Maly P (1989) Location of the mandibular canal: comparison of macroscopic findings, conventional radiography, and computed tomography. Int J Oral Maxillofac Implants 4: 327–332

Lam EW, Ruprecht A, Yang J (1995) Comparison of two-dimensional orthoradially reformatted computed tomography and panoramic radiography for dental implant treatment planning. J Prosthet Dent 74: 42–46

Lambrecht JTH (1995) 3-D modeling technology in oral and maxillofacial surgery. Chicago: Quintessence Publ Co Inc

Laney WR, Jemt T, Harris D, Henry PJ, Krogh PH, Polizzi G, Zarb GA, Herrmann I (1994) Osseointegrated implants for single-tooth replacement: progress report from a multicenter prospective study after 3 years. Int J Oral Maxillofac Implants 9: 49–54

Laney WR, Tolman DE (1989) The Mayo Clinic experience with tissue-integrated prostheses. In: Albrektsson T, Zarb GA, eds. The Brånemark osseointegrated implant. Chicago: Quintessence Publ Co Inc, pp 165–195

Larheim TA, Eggen S (1982) Measurements of alveolar bone height at tooth and implant abutments on intra-oral radiographs. A comparison of reproducibility of Eggen technique utilized with and without bite impression. J Clin Periodontol 9: 184–192

Ledermann PD (1989) ITI-Hohlzylinder nach 9 Jahren klinischer Erfahrung. Z Zahnärztl Implantol 5: 43–51

Lee S, Morgano SM (1994) A diagnostic stent for endosseous implants to improve conventional tomographic radiographs. J Prosthet Dent 71: 482–485

Lekholm U, van Steenberghe D, Herrmann I, Bolender C, Folmer T, Gunne J, Henry P, Higushi K, Laney WR, Lindén U (1994) Osseointegrated implants in the treatment of partially edentulous jaws: a prospective 5-year multicenter study. Int J Oral Maxillofac Implants 9: 627–635

Lekholm U, Zarb G (1985) Patient selection and preparation. In: Brånemark P-I, Zarb GA, Albrektsson T, eds. Tissue-integrated prostheses: osseointegration in clinical dentistry. Chicago: Quintessence Publ Co Inc, pp 199–209

Lekholm U, Adell R, Lindhe J, Brånemark P-I, Eriksson B, Rockler B, Lindvall AM, Yoneyama T (1986) Marginal tissue reactions at osseointegrated titanium fixtures. (II) A cross-sectional retrospective study. Int J Oral Maxillofac Surg 5: 53–61

Lima Verde MAR, Morgano SM (1993) A dual-purpose stent for the implant-supported prosthesis. J Prosthet Dent 69: 276–280

Lindh C, Petersson A, Klinge B (1992) Visualisation of the mandibular canal by different radiographic techniques. Clin Oral Impl Res 3: 90–97

Lindhe J, Berglundh T, Ericsson I, Liljenberg B, Marinello C (1992) Experimental breakdown of peri-implant and periodontal tissues. A study in the beagle dog. Clin Oral Impl Res 3: 9–16

Lindquist LW, Carlsson GE, Jemt T (1996) A prospective 15-year follow-up study of mandibular fixed prostheses supported by osseointegrated implants. Clinical results and marginal bone loss. Clin Oral Impl Res 7: 329–336

Lissac M, Coudert JL, Briguet A, Amiel M (1992) Disturbances caused by dental materials in Magnetic Resonance Imaging. Int Dent J 42: 229–233

Littner MM, Kaffe I, Arensburg B, Calderon S, Levin T (1995) Radiographic features of anterior buccal mandibular depression in modern human cadavers. Dentomaxillofac Radiol 24: 46–49

Luka B, Brechtelsbauer D, Gellrich N-C, König M (1995) 2D and 3D reconstructions of the facial skeleton: an unnecessary option or a diagnostic pearl? Int J Oral Maxillofac Surg 24: 76–83

Malmqvist JP, Sennerby L (1990) Clinical report on the success of 47 consecutively placed Core-Vent implants followed from 3 months to 4 years. Int J Oral Maxillofac Implants 5: 53–60

Marx RE, Johnson RP (1987) Studies in the radiobiology of osteoradionecrosis and their clinical significance. Oral Surg Oral Med Oral Pathol 64: 379–390

McKinney R, Koth D, Steflik D (1983) The single crystal sapphire endosseous dental implant. II. Two year results of clinical animal trials. J Oral Implantol 11: 629–637

Meidan Z, Weisman S, Baron J, Binderman I (1994) Technetium 99m-MDP scintigraphy of patients undergoing implant prosthetic procedures: a follow-up study. J Periodontol 65: 330–335

Meijer HJA, Steen WHA, Bosman F (1992) Aiming device for standardized intraoral radiographs of the alveolar crest around implants in the lower jaw. J Prosthet Dent 68: 318–321

Meijer HJA, Steen WHA, Bosman F (1993) A comparison of methods to assess marginal bone height around endosseous implants. J Clin Periodontol 20: 250–253

Merickse-Stern R, Steinlin Schaffner T, Marti P, Geering AH (1994) Peri-implant mucosal aspects of ITI implants supporting overdentures. A five-year longitudinal study. Clin Oral Impl Res 5: 9–18

Modica F, Fava C, Benech A, Preti G (1991) Radiologic-prosthetic planning of the surgical phase of the treatment of edentulism by osseointegrated implants: an in vitro study. J Prosthet Dent 65: 541–546

Molander B, Ahlqwist M, Gröndahl H-G (1995) Image quality in panoramic radiography. Dentomaxillofac Radiol 24: 17–22

Myers RA, Marx RE (1990) Use of hyperbaric oxygen in postradiation head and neck surgery. NCI-Monogr 151–157

Naert I, Quirynen M, van Steenberghe D, Darius P (1992) A six-year prosthodontic study of 509 consecutively inserted implants for the treatment of partial edentulism. J Prosthet Dent 67: 236–245

Nasr HF, Meffert RM (1993) A proposed radiographic index for assessment of the current status of osseointegration. Int J Oral Maxillofac Implants 8: 323–328

Nielsen IM, Glavind L, Karring T (1980) Interproximal periodontal intrabony defects. Prevalence, localization and etiological factors. J Clin Periodontol 7: 187–198

Nortje CJ, Farman AG, Grotepass FW (1977) Variations in the normal anatomy of the inferior dental (mandibular) canal: a retrospective study of panoramic radiographs from 3612 routine dental patients. Br J Oral Surg 15: 55–63

Petrikowski CG, Pharoah MJ, Schmitt A (1989) Presurgical radiographic assessment for implants. J Prosthet Dent 61: 59–64

Pharoah MJ (1993) Imaging techniques and their clinical significance. Int J Prosthodont 6: 176–179

Pilliar RM, Deporter DA, Watson PA, Valiquette N (1991) Dental implant design – effect on bone remodeling. J Biomed Mater Res 25: 467–483

Pitts NB (1984) Film holding, beam aiming and collimating devices as an aid to standardization in intraoral radiography. J Dent 12: 36–46

Powers MP, Bosker H, Van Pelt H, Dunbar N (1994) The transmandibular implant: from progressive bone loss to controlled bone growth. J Oral Maxillofac Surg 59: 904–910

Quirynen M, Lamoral Y, Dekeyser C, Peene P, van Steenberghe D, Bonte J, Baert AL (1990) The CT scan standard reconstruction technique for reliable jaw bone volume determination. Int J Oral Maxillofac Implants 5: 384–389

Quirynen M, Naert I, van Steenberghe D, Schepers E, Calberson L, Theuniers G, Ghyselen J, De Mars G (1991a) The cumulative failure rate of the Brånemark system in the overdenture, the fixed partial and the fixed full prosthesis design: A prospective study on 1237 fixtures. J Head Neck Pathol 10: 43–51

Quirynen M, van Steenberghe D, Jacobs R, Schotte A, Darius P (1991b) The reliability of pocket probing around screw-type implants. Clin Oral Impl Res 2: 186–192

Quirynen M, Naert I, van Steenberghe D, Duchateau L, Darius P (1992a) Periodontal aspects of Brånemark and IMZ implants supporting overdentures: a comparative study. In: Laney WR, Tolman DE, eds. Tissue integration in oral, orthopedic, maxillofacial reconstruction. Carol Stream (IL): Quintessence Publ Co Inc, pp 80–93

Quirynen M, Naert I, van Steenberghe D, Dekeyser C, Callens A (1992b) Periodontal aspects of osseointegrated fixtures supporting a partial bridge. J Clin Periodontol 19: 118–126

Quirynen M, Naert I, van Steenberghe D (1992c) Fixture design and overload influence marginal bone loss and fixture success in the Brånemark system. Clin Oral Impl Res 3: 104–111

Quirynen M, Naert I, van Steenberghe D (1992d) A study of 589 consecutive implants supporting complete fixed prostheses. Part I: Periodontal aspects. J Prosthet Dent 68: 655–663

Quirynen M, Naert I, van Steenberghe D (1993) Bacterial colonization of the internal part of two-stage implants. An in vivo study. Clin Oral Impl Res 4: 158–161

Rangert B (1993) Mechanical and biomechanical guidelines for the use of Brånemark System – general principles. Aust Prosthodont J 7(Suppl): 39–44

Ratliff F (1965) Mach bands: quantitative studies on neural networks in the retina. San Francisco: Holden-Day

Reddy MS, Mayfield-Donahoo TL, Jeffcoat MK (1992) A semi-automated computer assisted method for measuring bone support of dental implants. Clin Oral Impl Res 3: 28 – 31

Richter E-J, Jovanovic SA, Spiekermann H (1990) Rein implantatgetragene Brücken – eine Alternative zur Verbundbrücke? Z Zahnärztl Implantol VI: 137 – 144

Roberts WE, Simmons KE, Garetto LP, DeCastro RA (1992) Bone physiology and metabolism in dental implantology: risk factors for osteoporosis and other metabolic diseases. Implant Dent 1: 11 – 21

Rushton VE, Horner K (1996) The use of panoramic radiology in dental practice. J Dent 24: 185 – 201

Rydevik B, Brånemark P-I, Skalak R (1991) International workshop on osseointegration in skeletal reconstruction and joint replacement. Surte, Sweden: Minab, pp 11 – 16

Sanderink GC, Huiskens R, van der Stelt PF, Welander US, Stheeman SE (1994) Image quality of direct intraoral x-ray sensors in assessing root canal length. The radiovisiography, Visualix/Vix, Sens-A-Ray, and Flash Dent systems compared with Ektaspeed films. Oral Surg Oral Med Oral Pathol 78: 125 – 132

Schei O, Waerhaug J, Lovdal A, Arno A (1959) Alveolar bone loss as related to oral hygiene and age. J Periodontol 30: 7 – 16

Schnitman P, Rubenstein J, Jeffcoat M, Shulman L, Koch G (1980) Three-year survival results: blade implant versus cantilever clinical trial. J Dent Res 67: 1874

Schnitman PA, Schulman LB (1980) Dental implants: benefit and risk. An NIH-HARVARD Consensus Development Conference. Pub no. 81-1532. Bethesda. Department of Health and Human Services, National Institute of Health

Schramm-Scherer B, Behneke N, Reiber T, Tetsch P (1989) Röntgenologische Untersuchungen zur Belastung von Implantaten in zahnlosen Unterkiefer. Z Zahnärztl Implantol V: 185 – 190

Schwarz MS, Rothman SL, Chafetz N, Rhodes M (1989) Computed tomography in dental implantation surgery. Dent Clin North Am 33: 555 – 597

Sewerin I (1989) Radiographic control of fixture-abutment connection in Brånemark implant technique. Scand J Dent Res 97: 559 – 564

Sewerin I (1990) Errors in radiographic assessment of marginal bone height around osseointegrated implants. Scand J Dent Res 98: 428 – 433

Sewerin I (1991a) Estimation of angulation of Brånemark titanium fixtures from radiographic thread images. Clin Oral Impl Res 2: 20 – 23

Sewerin I (1991b) Comparison of radiographic image characteristics of Brånemark and IMZ implants. Clin Oral Impl Res 2: 151 – 156

Sewerin I (1991c) Tangential projection for depiction of the anterior regions of the jaws performed with the dental X-ray set. Tandlægebladet 95: 473 – 476

Sewerin I (1992) Radiographic image characteristics of Brånemark titanium fixtures. Swed Dent J 16: 7 – 12

Shapiro R (1972) Radiologic aspects of renal osteodystrophy. Radiol Clin North Am 3: 557 – 568

Shellock FG (1988) MR Imaging of metallic implants and materials: a compilation of the literature. Amer J Roentgenol. 151: 811 – 814

Simion M, Dahlin C, Trisi P, Piatelli A (1994) Qualitative and quantitative comparative study on different filling materials used in bone tissue regeneration: A controlled clinical study. Int J Periodontics Restorative Dent 14: 199 – 125

Smet M-H (1996) Three-dimensional skeletal visualisation with spiral computed tomography. Thesis, Catholic University Leuven

Smith DE, Zarb GA (1989) Criteria for success of osseointegrated endosseous implants. J Prosthet Dent 62: 567 – 572

Søballe K (1993) Hydroxyapatitie ceramic coating for bone implant fixation. Acta Orthop Scand (Suppl 255) 64: 1 – 58

Sonick M, Abrahams J, Faiella RA (1994) A comparison of the accuracy of periapical, panoramic and computerized tomographic radiographs in locating the mandibular canal. Int J Oral Maxillofac Implants 9: 455 – 460

Stella JP, Tharanon W (1990) A precise radiographic method to determine the location of the inferior alveolar canal in the posterior edentulous mandible: Implications for dental implants. Part 2: Clinical application. Int J Oral Maxillofac Implants 5: 23 – 29

Strid KG (1985a) Radiographic procedures. In: Brånemark P-I, Zarb GA, Albrektsson T, eds. Tissue-integrated prostheses: osseointegration in clinical dentistry. Chicago: Quintessence Publ Co Inc, pp 317 – 327

Strid KG (1985b) Radiographic results. In: Brånemark P-I, Zarb GA, Albrektsson T, eds. Tissue-integrated prostheses: osseointegration in clinical dentistry. Chicago: Quintessence Publ Co Inc, pp 187 – 198

Stromqvist B, Hansson L, Nilson L, Thorgren K (1987) Prognostic precision postoperative Tc-99m-MDP scintimetry after femoral neck fracture. Acta Orthop Scand 58: 494 – 498

Sundén S, Gröndahl H-G (1995) Accuracy and precision in the radiographic diagnosis of clinical instability in Brånemark dental implants. Clin Oral Impl Res 6: 220–226

Svenson B, Palmqvist S (1996) Imaging of dental implants in severely resorbed maxillae using detailed narrow-beam radiography. A methodological study. Dentomaxillofac Radiol 25: 67–70

Tammisalo E, Hallikainen D, Kanerva H, Tammisalo T (1992) Comprehensive oral X-ray diagnosis: Scanora multimodal radiography. A preliminary description. Dentomaxillofac Radiol 21: 9–15

Taylor TD, Worthington P (1993) Osseointegrated implant rehabilitation of the previously irradiated mandible: results of a limited trial at 3 to 7 years. J Prosthet Dent 69: 60–69

Teerlinck J, Quirynen M, Darius P, van Steenberghe D (1991) Periotest: an objective clinical diagnosis of bone apposition toward implants. Int J Oral Maxillofac Implants 6: 106–114

Todd AD, Gher ME, Quinetro G, Richardson AC (1993) Interpretation of linear and computed tomograms in the assessment of implant recipient sites. J Periodontol 64: 1243–1249

Tolman D, Keller E (1991) Endosseous implant placement immediately following dental extraction and alveoloplasty: preliminary report with 6-year follow-up. Int J Oral Maxillofac Implants 6: 24–28

Tricio J, Laohapand P-P, van Steenberghe D, Quirynen M, Naert I (1995) Mechanical state assessment of implant-bone continuum : a better understanding of the Periotest method. Int J Oral Maxillofac Implants 10: 43–49

Triplett RG, Schow SR (1996) Autologous bone grafts and endosseous implants: complementary techniques. J Oral Maxillofac Surg 54: 486–494

Trouerbach WT (1982) Radiographic aluminium equivalent value of bone. Thesis. Dordrecht: Van den Berg & Versluijs

Van Aken J (1969) Optimum conditions for intra-oral roentgenograms. Oral Surg Oral Med Oral Pathol 27: 75–91

Van den Akker HP (1988) Diagnostic imaging in salivary gland disease. Oral Surg 66: 625–637

Van der Stelt PF (1985) Experimentally produced bone lesions. Oral Surg Oral Med Oral Pathol 59: 306–312

Van der Velden U (1979) Probing force and the relationship of the probe tip to the periodontal tissues. J Clin Periodontol 6: 55–61

Van Drie HJY, Beertsen W, Grevers A (1988) Healing of the gingiva following instalment of Biotes implants in Beagle dogs. Adv Biomat 8: 485–490

van Steenberghe D, Lekholm U, Bolender C, Fohner C, Henry P, Herrmann I, Higuchi K, Laney W, Lindén U, Åstrand P (1990) The applicability of osseointegrated oral implants in the rehabilitation of partial edentulism: a prospective multicenter study on 558 fixtures. Int J Oral Maxillofac Implants 5: 272–281

van Steenberghe D, Brånemark P-I, Quirynen M, De Mars G, Naert I (1991) The rehabilitation of oral defects by osseointegrated implants. J Clin Periodontol 18: 488–493

van Steenberghe D, Klinge B, Linden U, Quirynen M, Herrmann I, Garpland C (1993) Periodontal indices around natural and titanium abutments: a longitudinal multicenter study. J Periodontol 64: 538–541

van Steenberghe D, Quirynen M (1993) Reproducibility and detection threshold of peri-implant diagnostics. Adv Dent Res 7: 191–195

van Steenberghe D, Tricio J, Naert I, Nys M (1995) Damping characteristics of bone-to-implant interfaces. Clin Oral Impl Res 6: 31–39

van Steenberghe D (1997) Outcomes and their treatment in clinical trials of endosseous oral implants. Ann Periodontol 2: 291–298

Van Waas MAJ (1983) Ridge resorption in denture wearers after vestibuloplasty and lowering of the floor of the mouth, measured on panoramic radiographs. Dentomaxillofac Radiol 12: 115–121

Versteegh PA, van Beeck GJ, Slagter AP, Ottervanger JP (1995) Clinical evaluation of mandibular overdentures supported by multiple-bar fabrication: a follow-up study of two implant systems. Int J Oral Maxillofac Implants 10: 595–603

Verstreken K, Van Cleynenbreugel J, Marchal G, Suetens P, Naert I, van Steenberghe D (1996) Computer assisted planning of oral implant surgery: a three-dimensional approach. Int J Oral Maxillofac Implants 11: 806–810

von Wowern N, Harder F, Hjørting-Hansen E, Gotfredsen K (1990) ITI implants with overdentures: a prevention of bone loss in edentulous mandibles? Int J Oral Maxillofac Implants 5: 135–139

von Wowern N (1985) Dual photon absorptiometry of mandibles: in vitro test of a new method. Scand J Dent Res 93: 167–177

von Wowern N, Kollerup G (1992) Symptomatic osteoporosis: a risk factor for reduction of the jaws. J Prosthet Dent 67: 656–660

von Wowern N, Storm TL, Olgaard K (1988) Bone mineral content by photon absorptiometry of the mandible compared with that of the forearm and the lumbar spine. Calcif Tissue Int 42: 157–161

Vos MH, Janssen PT, van Aken J, Heethaar RM (1986) Quantitative measurement of periodontal bone changes by digital subtraction. J Periodont Res 21: 583–591

Wagner A, Ploder O, Enislidis G, Truppe M, Ewers R (1995) Virtual image guided navigation in tumor surgery – technical innovation. J Craniomaxillofac Surg 23: 217–223

Webber RL, Rüttiman UE, Heaven TJ (1990) Calibration errors in digital subtraction radiography. J Periodont Res 25: 268–275

Weber HP, Buser D, Fiorellino JP, Williams RC (1992) Radiographic evaluation of crestal bone levels adjacent to nonsubmerged titanium implants. Clin Oral Impl Res 3: 181–188

Weiss MB, Ronen E (1977) New device to quantitative alveolar bone loss. Oral Surg Oral Med Oral Pathol 27: 106–110

Welander U, McDavid WD, Sanderink GC, Tronje G, Morner AC, Dove SB (1994) Resolution as defined by line spread and modulation transfer functions for four digital intraoral radiographic systems. Oral Surg Oral Med Oral Pathol 78: 109–115

Wenzel A (1989) Effect of manual compared with reference point superimposition on image quality in digital radiography. Dentomaxillofac Radiol 18: 145–150

Wenzel A (1993) Computer-aided image manipulation of intraoral radiographs to enhance diagnosis in dental practice: a review. Int Dent J 43: 99–108

White SC (1992) 1992 Assessment of radiation risk from dental radiography. Dentomaxillofac Radiol 21: 118–126

Wical KE, Swoope CC (1974) Studies on residual ridge resorption. Part I. Use of panoramic radiographs for evaluation and classification of mandibular resorption. J Prosthet Dent 32: 7–12

Wilding RJ, Slabbert JC, Kathree H, Owen CP, Crombie K, Delport P (1995) The use of fractal analysis to reveal remodelling in human alveolar bone following the placement of dental implants. Arch Oral Biol 40: 61–72

Wilson T Jr (1992) Guided tissue regeneration around dental implants in immediate and recent extraction sites: initial observations. Int J Periodontics Restorative Dent 12: 185–193

Witter PJ, Van Elteren P, Käyser AF, Van Rossum MJM (1989) The effect of removeable partial dentuses on the oral arches. J Oral Rehab 16: 27–33

World Workshop in Periodontics (1996) Consensus Report Implant therapy II. Annals Periodontol 1: 816–820

Yosue T, Brooks SL (1989a) The appearance of mental foramina on panoramic and periapical radiographs. II. Experimental evaluation. Oral Surg Oral Med Oral Pathol 68: 488–492

Yosue T, Brooks SL (1989b) The appearance of mental foramina on panoramic radiographs. I. Evaluation of patients. Oral Surg Oral Med Oral Pathol 68: 360–364

Zappa U, Simona C, Graf H, van Aken J (1991) In vivo determination of radiographic projection errors produced by a novel filmholder and an x-ray beam manipulator. J Periodontol 62: 674–683

Subject Index

Springer
and the
environment

At Springer we firmly believe that an
international science publisher has a
special obligation to the environment,
and our corporate policies consistently
reflect this conviction.
We also expect our business partners –
paper mills, printers, packaging
manufacturers, etc. – to commit
themselves to using materials and
production processes that do not harm
the environment. The paper in this
book is made from low- or no-chlorine
pulp and is acid free, in conformance
with international standards for paper
permanency.

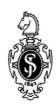

Springer

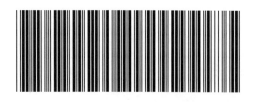